The Kidney at a Glance

The Kidney at a Glance

C.A. O'CALLAGHAN

BA, BM, BCh, MA, MRCP(UK), DPhil
MRC Clinician Scientist
Institute of Molecular Medicine
Nuffield Department of Medicine
University of Oxford
John Radcliffe Hospital
Oxford
UK

B.M. BRENNER

BS, MD, DM (Hon), DSc (Hon), FRCP
Samuel A. Levine Professor of Medicine
Havard Medical School and
Director, Renal Division
Brigham & Women's Hospital
Boston, MA
USA

Blackwell
Science

© 2000
Blackwell Science Ltd
Editorial Offices:
9600 Garsington Road
Oxford OX4 2DQ, UK
23 Ainslie Place, Edinburgh EH3 6AJ
350 Main Street, Malden
  MA 02148-5018, USA
54 University Street, Carlton
  Victoria 3053, Australia
10, rue Casimir Delavigne
  75006 Paris, France

Other Editorial Offices:
Blackwell Wissenschafts-Verlag GmbH
Kurfürstendamm 57
10707 Berlin, Germany

Blackwell Science KK
MG Kodenmacho Building
7–10 Kodenmacho Nihombashi
Chuo-ku, Tokyo 104, Japan

Iowa State University Press
A Blackwell Science Company
2121 S. State Avenue
Ames, Iowa 50014-8300, USA

The right of the Authors to be
identified as the Authors of this Work
has been asserted in accordance
with the Copyright, Designs and
Patents Act 1988.

First published 2000
Reprinted 2001
Reprinted 2003 (twice)

Set by Excel Typesetters Co., Hong Kong
Printed and bound in India
by Thomson Press (I) Ltd, India

The Blackwell Science logo is a
trade mark of Blackwell Science Ltd,
registered at the United Kingdom
Trade Marks Registry

DISTRIBUTORS
Marston Book Services Ltd
PO Box 269
Abingdon, Oxon OX14 4YN
(*Orders*: Tel: 01235 465500
         Fax: 01235 465555)

The Americas
Blackwell Publishing
c/o AIDC
PO Box 20
50 Winter Sport Lane
Williston, VT 05495-0020
(*Orders*: Tel: 800 216 2522
         Fax: 802 864 7626)

Australia
Blackwell Science Pty Ltd
54 University Street
Carlton, Victoria 3053
(*Orders*: Tel: 3 9347 0300
         Fax: 3 9347 5001)

A catalogue record for this title
is available from the British Library

ISBN 0-632-05206-6

Library of Congress
Cataloging-in-publication Data

O'Callaghan, C.A.
  The kidney at a glance/C.A. O'Callaghan, B.M. Brenner.
      p.   cm.
  Includes bibliographical references and index.
  ISBN 0-632-05206-6 (alk. paper)
  1. Kidneys—Diseases.   2. Kidneys.
  I. Brenner, Barry M., 1937–   II. Title.
  [DNLM: 1. Kidney Diseases—physiopathology.
  2. Kidney—physiology. WJ 300 O15k 2000]
  RC902 .O28 2000
  616.6′1—dc21
                                      00-028907

For further information on
Blackwell Science, visit our website:
www.blackwell-science.com

Contents

Preface

The last few years have seen huge advances in our understanding of how the kidney works and how abnormalities of renal function can affect the whole body. These developments have often resulted from the application of molecular biology which has led to the cloning of the major transport molecules, channels and receptors in the kidney, and from careful physiologic studies of the function of these molecules in health and disease. These advances in basic science have transformed the field into one that is highly rational and understandable at all levels from molecular studies of the transporter proteins, to clinical studies of patients. As an example, although drugs such as loop diuretics have been prescribed for many years, we now know the precise transporter molecules, which they inhibit and we can now teach, study and understand their actions on patients in a completely rational manner. Unfortunately, much of this new information has remained in specialist journals in a piecemeal fashion that makes it difficult for students or physicians to access or put into context.

Our intention is to bring this science in a clear manner to all who need to understand it. We believe that all medical students, doctors and other health-care providers need to understand the kidney, which is the site of action of so many commonly prescribed drugs and plays a key role in the pathophysiology of so many common disorders including congestive heart failure and hypertension. We have written this book to draw all this new information together and integrate it with the traditional concepts of renal function and disease. We hope that this new approach, which integrates all the relevant disciplines, including molecular biology, physiology and clinical medicine will be of use to all whose work involves the actions of the kidney. We believe that this applies to all students of medicine and all physicians. We also hope that this book will provide the information necessary for others, such as nurses, or non-clinical scientists to rapidly familiarize themselves with the parts of the subject which they need to know.

We have particularly emphasized an understanding of the normal mechanisms and the pathophysiology of the renal system. Although new drugs and treatments may be developed, they must act on the same systems and the same diseases, so a knowledge of basic renal function and pathophysiology will stand the reader in good stead for many years to come. This is an exciting field and to do it justice, we have set up a companion website which will provide a range of supplementary information, including updates on new developments in the field. The website also contains self-assessment material and keypoint summaries as well as suggestions for further reading and feedback. Do please visit the site at *www.learndoctor.com*.

We are very grateful to all at Blackwell Science for their enthusiasm and support; without them, this work would not have been possible. Lastly, we would like to thank our families for their support and all those who have kindly commented on the manuscript, especially Dr C.G. Winearls, Dr J.D. Firth and Dr R.M. Hilton. Their advice has been extremely helpful and any deficiencies that remain are entirely our own.

Chris O'Callaghan
Barry M. Brenner

Introduction and how to use this book

This book provides a comprehensive course in the major aspects of renal and urinary system science and disease, which is suitable for students of medicine and other life sciences. In addition, we hope that this book will be a valuable learning and revision tool for those in more advanced training and will provide a handy reference book for more experienced clinicians. In particular, the incorporation of the very latest molecular renal physiology makes this book ideal for those familiar with traditional renal science to update themselves with this new information.

Although most doctors are not renal physicians, the kidney is involved in many conditions. Almost all doctors prescribe drugs that act on the kidney, such as diuretics, on a regular basis, and are involved in assessing and adjusting fluid and electrolyte balance. For this reason, we believe that a clear understanding of renal science is essential for all who care for patients and we hope that this book provides the basis for such an understanding. As well as detailing specific renal diseases, there is full coverage of the major fluid and electrolyte disturbances.

We have placed a strong emphasis on the understanding of the mechanisms of disease because, unlike drugs or even clinical investigations, the mechanisms of a disease will be the same throughout a clinician's career. A good understanding of renal and electrolyte abnormalities will last a professional lifetime.

Renal science has undergone dramatic transformations over recent years, especially with the cloning of the major transporters and ion channels, and this makes the whole subject much easier to understand. We now know the precise molecular mechanisms of action of a number of key drugs, such as furosemide and the other diuretics, and it is now possible to give a clear explanation of their precise actions in a way that was not previously possible. We hope that readers and patients will benefit from an increased understanding of this subject.

The subject chapters are grouped into four sections and each chapter deals with a different topic. The first section provides a general introduction and essential background to the renal and urinary system; the second section deals with basic renal science; the third section deals with metabolic regulation and clinical disorders of fluid and electrolyte status; the fourth section deals with specific conditions affecting the kidney, with the common presentations of renal disease, and with approaches to the various modalities of acute and chronic renal replacement therapy. In general, each chapter is self-sufficient, but clearly cross-reference may be helpful. So, for example, it may be useful to review the chapters from the second section on renal sodium and water handling when studying the chapter in the third section on disorders of body sodium and water metabolism.

The individual chapters are arranged so that the essential material is encapsulated in the pictures, and in general it will not be necessary to try to memorize material that is not in the pictures. The text provides an explanation of the subject to accompany the pictures. We believe that, by giving a rational explanation of the subject matter, it should be easy to understand the material and subsequently to use the pictures as quick revision aids. Generally, if a subject is not understood properly it is very difficult to learn and the text should help learning by providing a rational explanation of all that is presented. Some readers find it helpful to add their own annotations to the pictures when studying or revising.

Several topics have been included for completeness and for more advanced readers, such as those training in internal medicine, pediatrics and nephrology or those aiming for particularly high marks in their examinations. A good example would be renal tubular acidosis.

Diagrams

The diagrams of ion movement are all drawn to the same style. In each case, the left side of the image and, therefore, of the cell, is the tubular lumen and the right side of the image and, therefore, of the cell, is the renal interstitium which leads on to the blood. In addition, transporter molecules are drawn as dark circles if they mediate active transport or as light circles if they mediate passive transport. Ion channels are shown as two straight lines (see Chapter 2).

Website

We have established a companion website for this book (*www.learndoctor.com*) and we encourage readers to explore this extra resource. It will provide updates on any major developments in the field and has a range of self-assessment material for each chapter, as well as detailed teaching answers, exploring issues raised in the chapters. In addition, there is further exploration of a number of more specialist topics or background information for those who are interested, as well as suggestions for further reading and useful links where appropriate. For rapid learning, we have also provided keypoint summaries for each chapter. We are particularly keen to get feedback from readers on this book and on our website and you can email any feedback or suggestions to the authors through the feedback link on the website or directly by email to *feedback@learndoctor.com*.

Abbreviations

ACE	angiotensin-converting enzyme
ACEI	angiotensin-converting enzyme inhibitor
AE	anion exchanger
AGBM	anti-glomerular basement membrane antibody
ANA	anti-nuclear antibody
ANCA	anti-neutrophil cytoplasmic antibody
ANP	atrial natriuretic peptide
ASOT/ASLO	anti-streptolysin O titre
ATP	adenosine triphosphate
BJP	Bence Jones protein
BUN	blood urea nitrogen
C4	a component of the alternative complement cascade
C3	a component of the common complement cascade, lowered by both classic and alternative complement activation
CRP	C-reactive protein
CT	computed tomography
DMSA	dimercaptosuccinic acid—used for radionuclide studies of renal function
dsDNA	double-stranded DNA
DTPA	diethylenetriaminepenta-acetic acid— used for radionuclide studies of renal perfusion
EDTA	ethylenediaminetetra-acetic acid
ESR	erythrocyte sedimentation rate
FF	filtration fraction
FMD	fibromuscular dysplasia
GBM	glomerular basement membrane
GFR	glomerular filtration rate
JGA	juxtaglomerular apparatus
MAG_3	mercaptoacetyl-triglycine
MR/MRI	magnetic resonance imaging
NHE	sodium/hydrogen (Na^+/H^+) exchanger
NSAIDs	non-steroidal anti-inflammatory drugs
PAH	p-aminohippurate
pH	negative logarithm of the hydrogen ion concentration
pK_a	the dissociation constant for an acid–base couple
RAS	renal artery stenosis
RBF	renal blood flow
RPF	renal plasma flow
RVH	renovascular hypertension

Glossary

Active transport. A transport process requiring energy in the form of ATP.

Aldosterone. A steroid produced by the adrenal cortex promoting sodium reabsorption in the collecting ducts.

Angiotensin II. A protein that is a potent vasoconstrictor; it acts via aldosterone and directly on the nephron to promote salt retention.

Antidiuretic hormone (ADH or vasopressin). A polypeptide produced by the posterior pituitary gland causing water reabsorption in the collecting duct.

Antiport. The same as counter transport.

Anuria. The complete absence of urine.

Apoptosis. Programmed cell death.

Atrial natriuretic peptide (ANP). A peptide produced by cardiac cells causing enhanced sodium excretion.

Bence Jones protein. Antibody light chains produced by B-cell dysplasias such as myeloma, which are present in the urine and may cause renal disease.

Bowman's capsule. The tubular epithelial component of the glomerulus which envelops the glomerular capillaries to form a space, Bowman's space, into which the filtrate passes.

Calyces. Divisions of the renal pelvis. The major calyces split into minor calyces and the renal papillae project into the minor calyces.

Carbonic anhydrase. An enzyme catalyzing the reaction of carbon dioxide and water.

Casts. Cylindrical aggregates of cells or protein debris formed in the distal tubules or collecting ducts.

Cloaca. The primitive excretory region in the fetus shared by both the urinary and gut drainage systems.

Collagen. A key protein in connective tissue.

Complement. A series of proteins triggered by infection or inflammation which promote tissue inflammation and destruction. C4 is a component of the alternative complement cascade. C3 is a component of the common complement cascade, lowered by both classic and alternative complement activation.

Cortex. The outer renal tissue containing the glomeruli and most of the proximal and distal tubules.

Co-transport. Transport of two molecules or ions in the same direction.

Counter-transport. Transport of two molecules or ions in opposite directions.

Creatine kinase. An enzyme released from damaged muscle.

Creatinine. A metabolic product of creatine metabolism filtered and secreted by the kidney.

Cytokines. Soluble molecules that can alter cellular behavior and attributes, particularly during inflammatory processes.

Doppler studies. Clinical studies that measure flow in vessels by the Doppler effect on ultrasound waves.

Efficacy. The effectiveness of treatment.

End-stage renal disease. A loss of renal function so severe that life cannot be maintained without renal replacement therapy.

Erythropoietin. A protein produced in the kidney which promotes red blood cell formation.

Fundoscopy. Looking at the retina, usually with an ophthalmoscope.

Glomerulonephritis. Disease of the glomeruli, usually with inflammation.

Hematocrit. The proportion of the blood that is made up of red blood cells.

Hematuria. Blood in the urine. Frank hematuria means visible blood in the urine.

Homeostasis. The maintenance of normal body conditions.

Hydrostatic pressure. The physical pressure of water—equivalent to hydraulic pressure.

Interstitial cells. Renal cells that support the matrix of the kidney but are not part of the nephron.

Interstitium. Connective tissue; in the kidney, the tissue that is not composed of vessels, nephrons, ducts, or other specialized components.

Inulin. A substance freely filtered but neither reabsorbed nor secreted, which can be used to estimate glomerular filtration rate.

Iso-osmotic. A process that occurs without causing a change in osmolality. Iso-osmotic reabsorption of sodium from the filtrate means that the sodium brings water with it, so that there is no overall change in the osmolality of the filtrate.

Juxtaglomerular apparatus (JGA). The combination of the tubular cells of the macula densa, granular afferent arteriolar cells that secrete renin, and extraglomerular mesangial cells.

Lateral. Away from the midline. Medial is towards the midline.

Macula densa. A patch of columnar tubular epithelial cells that forms part of the JGA and may sense tubular ion concentration. It is situated at the junction of the thick ascending limb of the loop of Henle and the early distal tubule.

Medial. Towards the midline. Lateral is away from the midline.

Medulla. The inner kidney constituting the renal pyramids and containing the loops of Henle, the medullary and papillary collecting ducts, and the vasa recta.

Mesangial cells. Renal cells in the glomerulus that support the glomerular capillary walls and may have some contractile function.

Mesonephric duct. The duct that forms the ejaculatory duct in men.

Mesonephros. The second fetal kidney.

Metanephros. The final fetal kidney which forms the adult kidney.

Myoglobin. A muscle protein with oxygen-binding capacity, which is toxic to renal tubules.

Myoglobinuria. Myoglobin in urine.

Nephritic syndrome. Acute glomerulonephritis with hypertension, renal impairment, and often edema.

Nephrolithiasis. The formation of renal stones.

Nephrocalcinosis. The diffuse deposition of calcium in the renal tissue.

Nephron. The basic excretory unit consisting of the glomerulus and its tubules.

Nephrotic syndrome. Proteinuria sufficient to cause a low serum albumin and peripheral edema.

Oncotic pressure. Colloid osmotic pressure.

Ontogeny. The pathway of cell differentiation.

Osmolality. The concentration of solutes in a given weight of water.

Osmosis. The movement of water through a semi-permeable membrane from a solution of low osmotic strength (low concentration) to one of high osmotic strength (high concentration).

Ostial lesion. Lesion at the opening of a vessel.

Papillary ducts. Ducts into which collecting ducts drain and which open out at the tip of the renal papilla into a minor calyx.

PAH. *p*-Aminohippurate: a substance completely cleared by a single pass through the kidney, which can be used to estimate renal blood flow.

Paramesonephric duct. The duct that forms the female reproductive tract.

Paraprotein. A protein that is present at high concentrations and is usually an antibody produced by a B-cell dysplasia, such as myeloma.

Parathyroid hormone. A protein produced by the parathyroid gland; it acts on the kidney to promote phosphate excretion, calcium reabsorption, and vitamin D production and it promotes calcium and phosphate release from bone.

Passive transport. A transport process that does not require energy.

Podocalyxin. A negatively charged glycoprotein that covers the pores in the glomerular capillary endothelial cells and forms part of the glomerular basement membrane.

Podocytes. The thin tubular epithelial cells which form part of the glomerular filtration barrier and cover the urinary aspect of the glomerular capillaries.

Polycythemia. Excess red blood cells in the blood.

Polyuria. Excess urine volume.

Polydipsia. Excess water intake.

Pontine myelinolysis. Destruction of tissue in the pons when there is rapid correction of disordered osmolality.

Pronephros. The earliest fetal kidney which is non-functional.

Renal hilus. The medial aspect of the kidney containing the entrance sites of the renal artery and vein and the renal pelvis.

Renal pelvis. The upper portion of the ureter leading into the calyces.

Renal replacement therapy. Treatment that takes over the function of the kidneys, usually dialysis, hemofiltration or transplantation.

Renin. An enzyme released by the JGA, which results in the formation of angiotensin II.

Reticulocyte. A nucleated red blood cell precursor.

Rhabdomyolysis. Muscle damage or destruction causing the release of nephrotoxic myoglobin.

Slit diaphragm. The tight junctions between adjacent podocytes which form part of the glomerular filtration barrier.

Tamm–Horsfall protein. A protein secreted by tubular cells, especially in the thick ascending limb of the loop of Henle. It helps to hold together casts which can form in the tubules.

Transepithelial gradient. An electrical or concentration gradient across the tubular epithelium.

Urea. A waste product of protein catabolism made by the liver and filtered and reabsorbed by the kidney.

Uricosuric. Causing uric acid excretion in the urine.

Vasa recta. Paired descending and ascending blood vessels which travel from the cortex to the medulla and back into the cortex with the loops of Henle.

Vasculitis. A disease process causing vessel inflammation and damage.

Vesical. Relating to the bladder, e.g. ureterovesical.

Vitamin D. A steroid hormone metabolized in the kidney to the active form 1,25-dihydroxycholecalciferol, which promotes calcium and phosphate absorption from the gut as a principal action.

Wolffian duct. The same as the mesonephric duct.

Nomenclature

USA and UK differences in spelling and nomenclature

The main differences relate to the use of 'ae' in the UK and 'e' in the USA.

USA	UK
anemia	anaemia
edema	oedema
hematocrit	haematocrit
hemoglobin	haemoglobin
hypercalcemia	hypercalcaemia
hyperkalemia	hyperkalaemia
hyponatremia	hyponatraemia
polycythemia	polycythaemia

In the USA, conventional units such as mg/dL are used, whereas in Europe and most other countries, the SI (Système International) units such as mmol/L are used. For creatinine, to convert from μmol/L to mg/dL divide by 88.4.

A number of terms differ, in particular:

USA	UK
cyclosporine	cyclosporin
epinephrine	adrenaline (although in the UK epinephrine is increasingly used)
furosemide	frusemide
vasopressin	antidiuretic hormone (ADH)

1 The kidney: structural overview

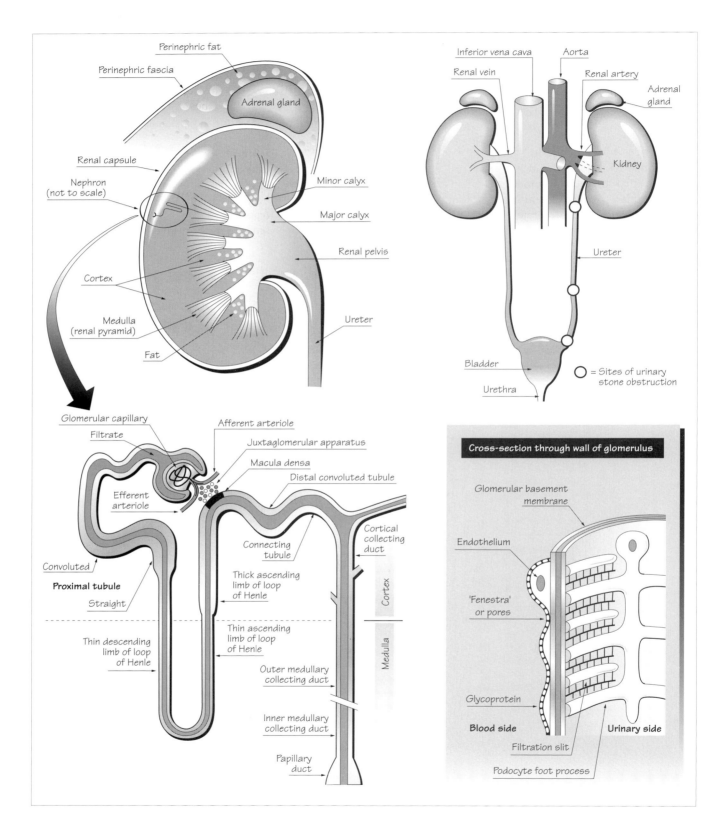

Gross anatomy

The kidney

The kidneys lie behind the peritoneum at the back of the abdominal cavity, extending from the twelfth thoracic vertebra (T12) to the third lumbar vertebra (L3). The right kidney is lower than the left because of the presence of the liver. During inspiration, both kidneys are pushed down as the diaphragm contracts. The kidney is covered by a fibrous capsule. This is further surrounded by perinephric fat and then by the perinephric (perirenal) fascia, which also enclose the adrenal gland. The renal cortex is the outer zone of the kidney and the renal medulla is the inner zone made up of the renal pyramids. The cortex contains all the glomeruli and the medulla contains the loops of Henle, the vasa recta, and the final portions of the collecting ducts.

Vessels and nerves

Blood vessels and the ureter connect with the kidney at the renal hilus. The renal artery arises from the aorta and usually divides into three branches. Two pass in front of the ureter and one goes behind it. Five or six small veins come together to form the renal vein, which leaves the kidney in front of the anterior branch of the renal artery and enters the inferior vena cava. The position of the lymphatics and the renal sympathetic nerves is variable. The lymphatics drain to the lateral aortic lymph nodes. Sympathetic nerves supply the renal vasculature and juxtaglomerular apparatus, and to a lesser extent the rest of the nephron. Afferent fibers enter the spinal cord at T10, T11, and T12.

The draining system for urine

Within the kidney, the pelvis of the ureter divides into two or three major calyces, each of which subdivides into two or three minor calyces. Each minor calyx contains a renal papilla which is the apex of a medullary pyramid. The ureter passes out of the kidney behind the peritoneum on the psoas muscle and then enters the pelvis in front of the sacroiliac joint. It moves down the lateral pelvic wall towards the ischial spine and then turns forward and medially to enter the bladder. It passes through the bladder wall for 2 cm before opening into the bladder. Urine passes along the ureter by peristalsis. The ureter has three constrictions where kidney stones can become lodged (see Chapter 47). Afferent nerves from the ureter enter the spinal cord at T11, T12, L1, and L2. The bladder is innervated by S3, S4, and S5.

Microanatomy

The nephron

The nephron is the basic unit of the kidney. Each kidney has 400 000–800 000 nephrons, although this number falls with age. A nephron consists of the glomerulus and the associated tubule that leads to the collecting duct. Urine is formed by filtration in the glomerulus; it is then modified in the tubules by reabsorption and secretion of substances. Cortical nephrons occur throughout the renal cortex and have short loops of Henle; juxtamedullary nephrons begin near the corticomedullary junction and have long loops of Henle, which descend deep into the medulla and enable them to concentrate urine effectively. Cortical nephrons outnumber juxtamedullary nephrons by 7:1.

Interstitial cells in the kidney

The cortex contains two types of interstitial cell: phagocytic and fibroblast-like cells. Erythropoietin is made in the fibroblast-like cells. Three types of medullary interstitial cells have been identified. One type contains lipid droplets which may provide precursors for synthesis of prostaglandin in the kidneys.

The glomerulus as a filtration barrier

The glomerulus is a ball of capillaries surrounded by the Bowman's capsule, a hollow capsule of the tubular epithelium into which urine is filtered. The glomerulus also contains mesangial cells, which provide a scaffold to support capillary loops and have contractile and phagocytic properties. Blood enters the glomerular capillaries from an afferent arteriole and leaves through an efferent arteriole, rather than a venule. Vasoconstriction of this efferent arteriole creates a high hydrostatic pressure in the glomerular capillary, forcing water, ions, and small molecules through the filtration barrier into Bowman's capsule. Whether a substance is filtered depends on both its molecular size and charge. The filtration barrier has three layers:

1 *Endothelial cells.* The endothelial cells of the glomerular capillary wall are thin, with numerous 70-nm pores filled with negatively charged glycoprotein, mostly podocalyxin.

2 *Glomerular basement membrane.* This specialized capillary basement membrane also contains negatively charged glycoproteins. It has two layers, made up of type IV collagen, heparan sulfate proteoglycans, laminin, podocalyxin and low levels of type III and V collagen, fibronectin, and entactin. Type IV collagen forms helical strands which are arranged into a three-dimensional framework on to which the other components are attached.

3 *Epithelial cells of Bowman's capsule.* The epithelial cells or podocytes have long projections from which foot processes arise and attach to the urinary side of the glomerular basement membrane. Foot processes from different podocytes interdigitate, leaving filtration slits of 25–65 nm between them. Across these slits, a highly organized network of several glycoproteins forms 'slit pores' through which filtration occurs and which prevent the passage of larger molecules such as albumin.

2 The kidney: functional overview

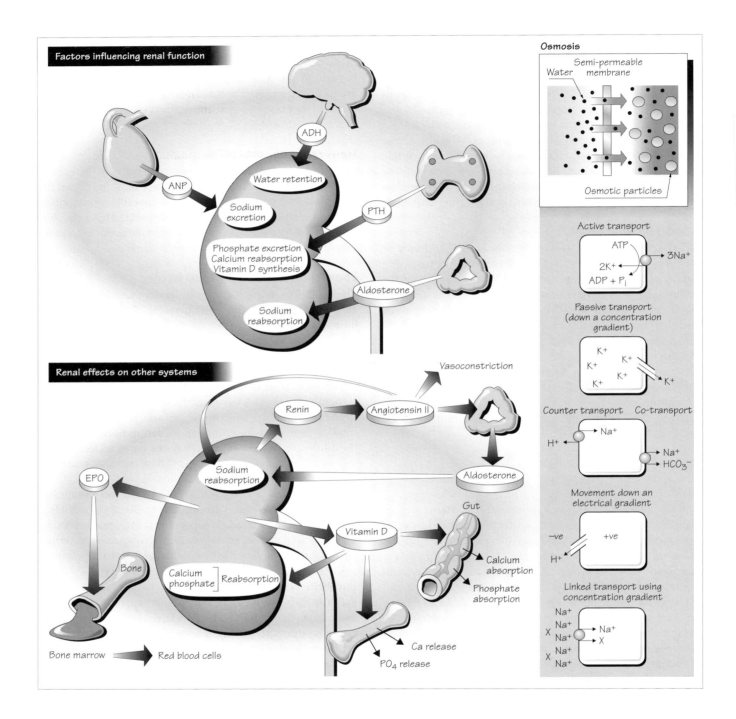

The kidney maintains a stable extracellular environment which supports the function of all body cells. It controls water and ionic balance by regulating the excretion of water, sodium, potassium, chloride, calcium, magnesium, phosphate, and many other substances, and by managing acid–base status.

Tubular function

The urinary filtrate formed in the glomerulus passes into the tubules where its volume and content are altered by reabsorption or secretion. Most solute reabsorption occurs in the proximal tubules, with fine adjustments to urine composition being made in the distal tubule and collecting ducts. The loop of Henle serves to concentrate urine.

The tubular epithelium is only one cell thick. Tubular cells have tight junctions at their apical or luminal edges which separate tubular fluid from peritubular plasma, allowing transport processes to establish concentration gradients across the tubular epithelium. In Bowman's capsule the cells are thin squamous epithelial cells, but in the tubules the cells are mainly columnar epithelial cells designed for transport processes.

Proximal tubule
The proximal tubule is initially convoluted and then straightens out as it leads down to the loop of Henle. The tubular cells are tall, columnar epithelial cells with many microvilli, a high surface area, and a well-developed luminal endocytic apparatus. Many substances are actively reabsorbed in the proximal tubule, including sodium, potassium, calcium, phosphate, glucose, amino acids, and water. This reabsorption reduces the volume of filtrate but, because water moves osmotically with the reabsorbed solutes, the filtrate is not concentrated (i.e. iso-osmotic reabsorption).

Loop of Henle
As the straight proximal tubule becomes the thin descending limb of the loop of Henle, the cells become flatter with fewer microvilli. Next comes the thin ascending limb, followed by the thick ascending limb, which contains predominantly cuboidal cells. The thick ascending limb passes up toward the glomerulus from which it arose, ending at the macula densa.

Juxtaglomerular apparatus
The juxtaglomerular apparatus is a compound structure that consists of a patch of tubular cells termed the **macula densa**, granular cells mainly in the afferent arteriolar wall, and extraglomerular mesangial cells. The granular cells in the arterioles secrete renin (see Chapter 13).

Distal tubule
Beyond the macula densa is the distal convoluted tubule. This leads to the collecting tubule which drains into the collecting duct. The collecting duct has three sections, named according to their depth in the kidney: the cortical collecting duct, the outer medullary collecting duct, and the inner medullary collecting duct. The inner medullary collecting duct flows into a papillary duct, which opens out on a renal papilla into a minor calyx.

Blood vessels associated with the loop of Henle
The efferent arterioles in cortical nephrons form a second capillary bed, the peritubular capillaries, which surrounds the rest of the tubular system. However, in the juxtamedullary nephrons, the efferent arterioles first form vascular bundles that give rise to both the peritubular capillaries and the straight vessels, which in turn form the vasa recta. The descending vasa recta go down into the inner medulla with the loop of Henle. At this level, the vessel branches to form a capillary network, which leads on to the ascending vasa recta. These veins travel upwards in close proximity to the descending vasa recta. The vasa recta are the sole blood supply to the medulla (see Chapter 11).

Transport processes in the tubules
Active transport requires energy expenditure in the form of ATP (e.g. $3Na^+/2K^+$ ATPase). Ions or molecules can move by *passive transport* down an electrical or concentration gradient. Water molecules cannot be pumped directly; they move by *osmosis* when there is a concentration gradient of ions or molecules across a semipermeable membrane. If charged particles are moved, electroneutrality is maintained either by *co-transport* in the same direction of a particle of opposite charge or by *counter-transport* in the opposite direction of a particle of the same charge. Molecules can move by *linked transport* to another molecule which is moving down an electrical or concentration gradient.

Hormones acting on the kidney
- **Antidiuretic hormone (ADH or vasopressin).** This is a peptide released by the posterior pituitary gland; it promotes water reabsorption in the collecting ducts.
- **Aldosterone.** This is a steroid hormone produced by the adrenal cortex; it promotes sodium reabsorption in the collecting ducts.
- **Atrial natriuretic peptide.** This is produced by cardiac cells; it promotes sodium excretion in the collecting ducts.
- **Parathyroid hormone.** This is a protein produced by the parathyroid gland; it promotes renal phosphate excretion, calcium reabsorption and vitamin D production.

Hormones produced by the kidney
- **Renin.** This is a protein released by the juxtaglomerular apparatus; it results in the formation of *angiotensin II*, which acts directly on the nephron and via aldosterone to promote sodium retention, and which is also a potent vasoconstrictor.
- **Vitamin D.** This is a steroid hormone metabolized in the kidney to the active form 1,25-dihydroxycholecalciferol, which promotes calcium and phosphate absorption from the gut as a principal action.
- **Erythropoietin.** This is a protein produced in the kidney; it promotes red blood cell formation in bone marrow.
- **Prostaglandins.** These are produced in the kidney; they have various effects, especially on renal vessel tone.

3 Development of the renal system

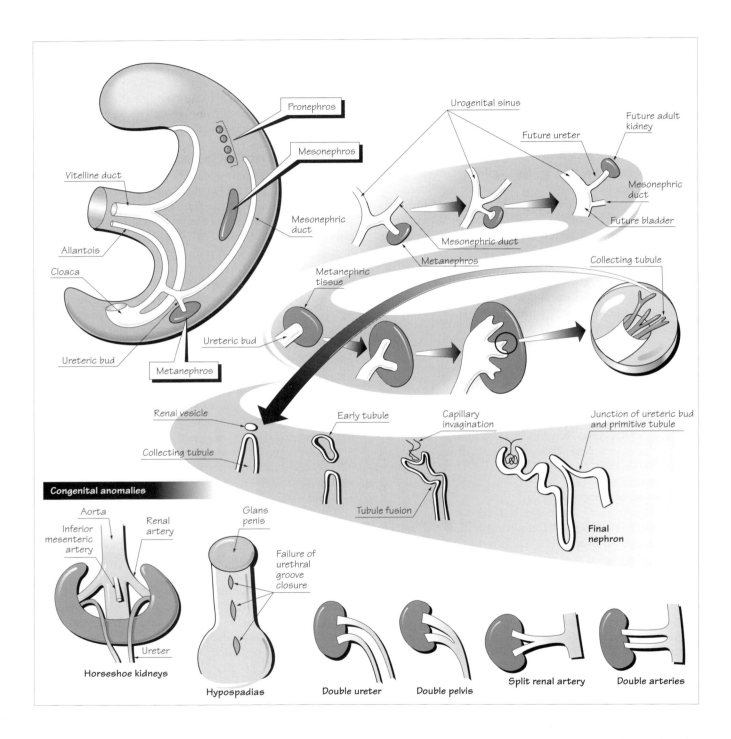

The renal and genital systems both develop from the intermediate mesoderm, a collection of cells at the back of the fetal abdominal cavity. Both systems initially drain into the same space, the fetal cloaca. During development, the intermediate mesoderm first forms the pronephros in the cervical region, second the mesonephros below this, and last the metanephros in the pelvic region. The pronephros and mesonephros regress and do not form part of the adult kidney. The metanephros forms the final adult kidney and becomes functional in the second half of the pregnancy.

Although the fetus swallows amniotic fluid, digests it, and excretes urine into the amniotic fluid, it is the placenta that removes fetal waste products for excretion by the mother's kidneys.

The development of all three kidney systems requires the induction of mesenchyme to become epithelium. In the metanephros, the ureteric bud induces mesenchyme around its tips to form nephrons. This metanephric mesenchyme forms the tubular system from the glomerulus to the distal nephron, whereas the ureteric bud forms the collecting duct and draining system.

Kidney formation in detail

Around week 4 of gestation, clusters of cells in the intermediate mesoderm form very primitive glomeruli in the cervical region. Together, these form the non-functional pronephros which later regresses. However, the lateral portions of the cell clusters at each level fuse to form the mesonephric (or Wolffian) duct, which grows downwards and enters the cloaca. As the pronephros regresses, the intermediate mesoderm below it forms the mesonephros. This may function briefly, draining into the mesonephric duct, but it regresses by the end of the second month.

Nephron formation in the metanephros

From week 5 onwards, the metanephros forms from intermediate mesoderm cells in the pelvis. Just above the entrance of the mesonephric duct into the cloaca, an outgrowth of the duct called the ureteric bud invades the metanephric tissue mass. The bud dilates to form the renal pelvis, splits progressively to form the calyces, and then small branches elongate to form the collecting tubules. Metanephric tissue at the tips of these collecting ducts aggregates and forms vesicles that develop into tubules. Capillaries invaginate one end of each tubule to form a glomerulus. The newly formed tubule lengthens to form the proximal tubule, loop of Henle, and distal tubule. At the other end, the tubule connects to the collecting tubule that induced its formation.

Renal position and congenital anomalies

In the pelvis, the metanephric kidney receives its blood supply from pelvic branches of the aorta. As the kidneys move upwards to their final posterior abdominal position, these original arteries regress and the kidneys are vascularized by the renal arteries which come off the aorta at a higher level. It is common for some of the earlier arteries to persist as supernumerary renal arteries. It is also possible for one or both kidneys to remain permanently in the pelvis. If both kidneys stay in the pelvis, they can be forced together and fuse at the lower poles to form a horseshoe kidney, which cannot then rise because of the inferior mesenteric artery above it. If the ureteric bud splits early, the result can be two ureters or two renal pelvices connecting to one ureter.

Bladder and urethra formation

The cloaca is split by a septum into a posterior anorectal region and an anterior urogenital sinus. The ureteric buds form the ureters which drain into the mesonephric ducts; these then drain into the urogenital sinus. The lower part of the mesonephric ducts becomes absorbed into the wall of the urogenital sinus to form the trigone area of the bladder. This means that, eventually, the mesonephric ducts and the ureters enter the sinus separately. As the kidneys ascend, the openings of the ureters move up the urogenital sinus into the zone that they will occupy when that part of the urogenital sinus becomes the bladder. The lower part of the urogenital sinus forms part of the urethra in both sexes and, in females, it also forms part of the vestibule. In males, the mesonephric ducts form the ejaculatory ducts. A paramesonephric duct also forms and, in females, develops into much of the female upper reproductive tract.

On either side of the anterior cloaca, swellings form into urethral folds which meet above the cloaca as a genital tubercle. In females, the urethral folds develop into the labia minora. In males, this grows to form a phallus, pulling the urethral folds along to form the lateral walls of a groove below the future glans penis. The folds close over to form the penile urethra. Incomplete fusion of the folds causes hypospadias with a urethral opening along the inferior aspect of the penis. The final distal part of the male urethra is formed by an ingrowth of cells which form the external urethral meatus.

Molecules implicated in renal development

WT-1, the Wilms' tumor gene-1, is a transcription factor expressed at high levels in metanephric mesenchyme (see Chapter 48). In WT-1 knockout mice, no metanephric kidney or gonads form. N-myc, a proto-oncogene, and the transcription factors Pax2 and Pax8 are all expressed in the developing metanephric kidney. Other molecules that may play a role in metanephric development include the oncogene bcl-2, a secreted glycoprotein Wnt-4, a TGFβ (transforming growth factor β) family molecule OP-1, the PDGF (platelet-derived growth factor) family proteins, and the c-Ret tyrosine kinase. Abnormalities produced by polycystic kidney disease genes are considered in Chapter 38.

4 Clinical features of kidney disease

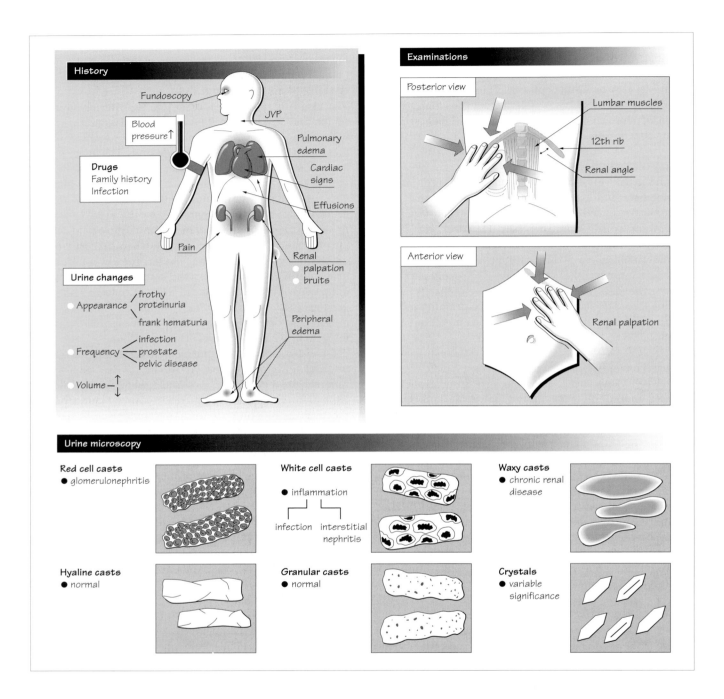

There are more nephrons in each kidney than are needed to sustain life and so kidney disease may not become clinically apparent until there is substantial loss of renal function. For this reason, slowly progressive renal diseases can be asymptomatic in the early stages.

History

Pain

Pain is uncommon with renal disease, but can occur if there is urinary obstruction, especially from renal stones. Infection or distention of the renal capsule or of renal cysts, especially in polycystic kidney disease, can also cause pain.

Inflammation of the bladder or urethra, usually as a result of infection, can cause dysuria (discomfort on micturition). Rarely, glomerular disease can cause a dull lumbar ache.

Urine appearance and volume

Proteinuria can produce frothy urine and frank *hematuria* is obvious as red or pink urine. Dark urine can also occur with the myoglobinuria of rhabdomyolysis or the hemoglobinuria of hemolysis. Recurrent intermittent frank hematuria suggests immunoglobulin A (IgA) glomerulonephritis in young people or renal tract cancer in elderly people. Glomerular bleeding is present throughout the stream, whereas hematuria only at the beginning of the stream suggests urethral bleeding and hematuria only late in the stream suggests bladder or prostate bleeding.

Increased urinary frequency is an increase in the frequency of micturition. Polyuria is an increase in total urine volume. Increased *urinary frequency*, especially at night, can suggest prostatic enlargement in men or urinary tract infection. *Polyuria* suggests a defect of renal urine-concentrating mechanisms or excess water ingestion. Prostatic enlargement can also cause hesitancy and terminal dribbling as well as obstruction and urinary retention. Total *anuria* is rare and usually suggests urethral or bilateral ureteric obstruction, a severe rapidly progressive glomerulonephritis, or aortic or bilateral renal arterial occlusion.

General history

Always take a full history. Establish whether the patient has a previous history of hypertension, diabetes mellitus, malignancy, or other systemic diseases. Any recent infection, but typically a streptococcal throat infection, can trigger a postinfective glomerulonephritis. The drug history may indicate use of nephrotoxic drugs, especially analgesics or nonsteroidal anti-inflammatory drugs. A family history of renal disease can suggest a hereditary disorder, especially polycystic kidney disease. Symptoms of itching, muscle cramps, anorexia, nausea, and even confusion are consistent with chronic renal impairment. Hemoptysis suggests a vasculitic disease, particularly Goodpasture's syndrome.

Examination

Carry out a full examination including blood pressure measurement, fundoscopy, examination for edema, and rectal and vaginal examinations where appropriate. Check for a distended bladder. Look for signs of systemic disease in all systems, especially neurologic and rheumatologic signs. Cardiac valve lesions raise the possibility of glomerulonephritis associated with infective endocarditis. Peripheral bruits or absent peripheral pulses indicate vascular disease and such patients are at risk of renal artery stenosis, which may result in renal artery bruits.

Kidneys

Enlarged kidneys may be palpable. The right kidney, which lies lower than the left because of the liver, is sometimes palpable when normal. To palpate the kidneys, place the right hand over the upper abdomen on the relevant side. On the same side, place the left hand with the fingers in the renal angle formed by the lateral margin of the lumbar muscles and the twelfth rib. As the patient inspires, push the fingers of the left hand anteriorly several times. You will feel an enlarged kidney with the right hand as it moves down the abdominal cavity during inspiration and is pushed anteriorly by the fingers of your left hand.

Fluid status

It is important to determine whether the patient has an excess or a deficiency of body water. Useful physical signs to look for include peripheral pitting edema, detectable especially at the ankles and sacrum, signs of pulmonary edema, effusions, the jugular venous pulse pressure, and skin turgor. A cardiac gallop rhythm may suggest hypervolemia. A low blood pressure, especially with a postural drop, indicates hypovolemia.

Bedside investigation of urine

Dipstick test urine for hematuria, proteinuria, and glucosuria. Use a microscope, ideally with phase contrast, to examine fresh urine. If possible, centrifuge the urine and discard most of the supernatant to concentrate cells or casts.

Red cells. These can arise from anywhere in the urinary tract, but deformed red cells indicate glomerular bleeding.

White cells. These suggest inflammation, resulting from bacterial infection if they are polymorphonuclear cells or interstitial nephritis if they are eosinophils or lymphocytes.

Casts. These are cylindrical aggregates formed in the distal tubule or collecting ducts. *Hyaline casts* and fine *granular casts* are normal findings. Hyaline casts are mainly protein and may be increased in proteinuria. Granular casts are also mainly protein. *Fatty casts* can occur in the nephrotic syndrome. *Waxy casts* are large and occur in dilated tubules in chronic renal failure. *Red cell casts* indicate glomerular bleeding, usually due to glomerulonephritis. *White cell casts* suggest acute infection, usually bacterial.

Crystals. These may indicate a stone-forming tendency, but are not always of pathologic significance because they can form after urine collection. Ideally, examine urine for crystals when it is fresh and at 37 °C.

Infectious agents. Take a midstream urine sample for culture. Nitrites on dipstick analysis suggest infection.

Proteinuria. Quantify any proteinuria by measuring the amount of protein in a 24-h urine collection.

5 The kidney: laboratory investigations and diagnostic imaging

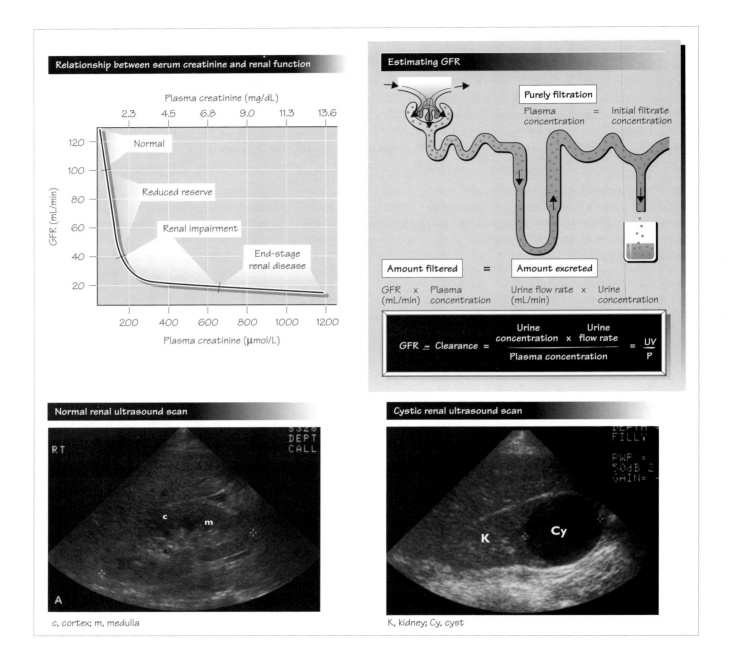

Relationship between serum creatinine and renal function

Plasma creatinine (mg/dL)

Normal

Reduced reserve

Renal impairment

End-stage renal disease

Plasma creatinine (μmol/L)

Estimating GFR

Purely filtration

Plasma concentration = Initial filtrate concentration

Amount filtered = Amount excreted

GFR (mL/min) × Plasma concentration   Urine flow rate (mL/min) × Urine concentration

$$GFR \approx Clearance = \frac{Urine\ concentration \times Urine\ flow\ rate}{Plasma\ concentration} = \frac{UV}{P}$$

Normal renal ultrasound scan

c, cortex; m, medulla

Cystic renal ultrasound scan

K, kidney; Cy, cyst

Blood tests

Take venous blood for routine biochemistry and hematology. A priority is to check that the serum potassium level is not dangerously elevated.

Estimating the glomerular filtration rate
Serum urea and creatinine

As urea and creatinine are excreted by the kidneys, they accumulate in the blood when renal function is impaired. However, because there is excess renal capacity, neither substance rises substantially until the glomerular filtration rate (GFR) falls to around 30 mL/min from a normal value of around 120 mL/min. **Urea** levels rise with a high protein intake or a catabolic state and fall with liver disease or overhydration. Urea is freely filtered, but there is also some tubular reabsorption which is increased (along with sodium

ducts, to maintain accurate salt balance. About 5% of the salt intake is lost in sweat and feces.

The basolateral membranes of the tubular cells contain Na^+/K^+ ATPases that actively pump sodium into the peritubular plasma. From here, sodium ions pass freely into the blood to complete the reabsorption process. The continual pumping of sodium out of the cells and its subsequent removal by the blood creates a Na^+ gradient between the tubular filtrate and the cell cytoplasm. This gradient allows Na^+ from the filtrate to enter the cells passively at their apical membrane, provided that suitable channels or transporters are present.

Sodium handling along the nephron
Proximal tubule
Of the filtered sodium, 65% is reabsorbed in the proximal tubule. In the early proximal tubule, a large amount of reabsorption takes place, but the cell junctions are slightly leaky, limiting the concentration gradient that can be established between the filtrate and the peritubular plasma. In the late proximal tubule, the transport rate is lower, but tight junctions allow a larger gradient to be established.

In the early tubule, the sodium gradient drives the co-transport of sodium with bicarbonate, amino acids, glucose, or other organic molecules. The Na^+/H^+ exchanger (NHE-3) uses the sodium gradient to drive sodium reabsorption from the filtrate and H^+ secretion into the filtrate. As carbonic anhydrase is present in the cell cytoplasm and tubular lumen, the secretion of H^+ is equivalent to the reabsorption of bicarbonate (HCO_3^-) (see Chapters 8 and 9). The apical secretion of H^+ is balanced by the basolateral exit of bicarbonate with sodium. When the positively charged sodium ions leave the lumen with neutral organic molecules, the lumen is left with a negative charge. This repels negatively charged chloride ions, which leave the lumen through the paracellular route between the cells.

By the time the filtrate reaches the late proximal tubule, most organic molecules and bicarbonate have already been removed and sodium ions are reabsorbed mainly with chloride ions. The Na^+/H^+ exchanger works in parallel to a chloride/base exchanger and, as the base—usually formate, oxalate, or bicarbonate is recycled across the apical membrane—the overall effect is that sodium chloride is reabsorbed. Chloride ions leave the cell alone or in exchange for another negatively charged ion or in co-transport with potassium.

The loop of Henle
The thin and thick ascending portions of the loop of Henle together reabsorb 25% of the filtered sodium.

Thin segments
Cells in the walls of the thin segments of the loop are thin and flat epithelial cells. No active transport occurs here and there are few mitochondria. The thin descending segment is permeable to water but not to sodium, so water leaves the tubule passively to enter the hypertonic medullary interstitium. In contrast, the thin ascending limb is permeable to sodium but not to water. As the filtrate loses water in the descending limb, there is a high concentration of sodium and chloride ions in the lumen of the thin ascending limb, and both ions diffuse out.

Thick ascending limb
The cells of the thick segment of the loop are large, with multiple mitochondria that generate energy for the active transport of sodium ions.

The key transport molecule is the NaK2Cl transporter which uses the sodium gradient for the co-transport of two chloride ions with one sodium and one potassium ion. As the potassium ion can re-enter the tubule via the ROMK channel, the net effect is the removal of one sodium and two chloride ions, leaving the tubular lumen positively charged. This positive potential drives the paracellular transport of positively charged ions, including sodium, potassium, calcium, magnesium and ammonium. The NaK2Cl transporter has multiple transmembrane domains and is inhibited by the diuretic furosemide (see Chapter 15).

Distal tubule
The distal tubule reabsorbs a further 5% of the filtered sodium. This transport occurs via a sodium chloride co-transport protein that is inhibited by the thiazide diuretics. As the fluid in the lumen in this portion of the nephron is negative, there is also some paracellular movement of negatively charged chloride ions.

Collecting tubules and ducts
Around 2–5% of filtered sodium is reabsorbed in the collecting ducts, which contain two characteristic cell types.
- **The principal cells.** Sodium enters these cells via the epithelial sodium channel (ENaC), leaving the lumen negatively charged. This negative charge drives the paracellular movement of chloride. The ENaC channel is composed of three homologous subunits and is inhibited by the diuretic drug amiloride.
- **The intercalated cells.** These have no Na^+/K^+ ATPase but do have an H^+ ATPase, which establishes a hydrogen ion gradient. The energy required for the transport function of these cells is derived from this H^+ gradient instead of the usual Na^+ gradient. As H^+ ions are removed from the cell, the net result is the secretion of bicarbonate coupled to the reabsorption of chloride.

Chloride reabsorption by the intercalated cells and sodium reabsorption by principal cells are the final stage in sodium chloride reabsorption before urine leaves the kidney.

7 Renal potassium handling

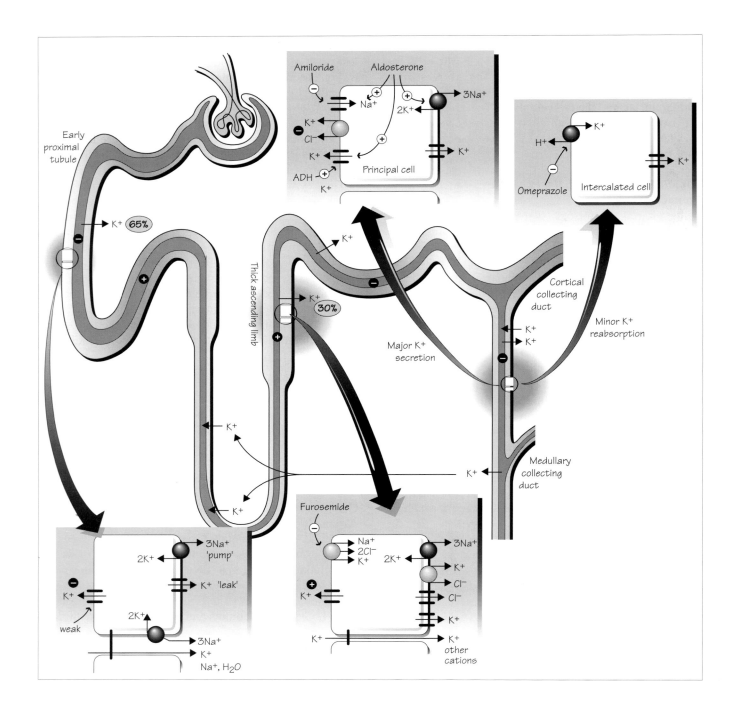

Potassium is the major intracellular cation. The potassium concentration inside cells is around 150 mmol/L, compared with around 4 mmol/L in extracellular fluid. The K⁺ gradient across the cell membrane largely determines the electrical potential across that membrane. As this electrical potential influences the electrical excitability of tissues such as nerves and muscles, including the cardiac muscle, potassium levels must be precisely controlled within safe limits.

The average daily intake of potassium in the diet is around 40–120 mmol, but the kidneys filter around 800 mmol each day. To maintain potassium balance, the kidney therefore excretes only 5–15% of the filtered potassium. Potassium, like sodium, is freely filtered in the glomerulus, but is handled quite differently in the tubules. Sodium ions are reabsorbed throughout the nephron, and any sodium that is excreted is simply that which has not been reabsorbed. In contrast, almost all the filtered potassium is reabsorbed before the filtrate reaches collecting tubules. *Potassium that is to be excreted is then secreted into the collecting duct.*

Only 2% of the total body potassium is outside cells in the extracellular fluid and, in order to maintain appropriate intracellular potassium concentrations, all cells use a **pump-leak** mechanism. This consists of the Na^+/K^+ ATPase pump, which actively transports potassium into the cell, balanced by various channels, which allow potassium to leak out of the cell. Intracellular potassium can be controlled by changing the activity of the pump or by altering the number or the permeability of the potassium channels. In tubular cells, the cell membrane is divided into apical and basolateral portions, each of which has different populations of pumps and channels. This allows the pump-leak system to be used to transport potassium across the tubular epithelium. As with sodium handling, the major driving force behind potassium movement is the Na^+/K^+ ATPase.

Potassium handling along the nephron
Proximal tubule
Of the filtered potassium ions, 65% are reabsorbed in the proximal tubule. No specific potassium channels for this reabsorption have been identified. Potassium reabsorption is tightly linked to that of sodium and water, with similar proportions of the filtered sodium, water, and potassium being reabsorbed in this segment. The reabsorption of sodium drives that of water which may carry some potassium with it. The potassium gradient resulting from the reabsorption of water from the tubular lumen drives the paracellular reabsorption of potassium and may be enhanced by the removal of potassium from the paracellular space via the Na^+/K^+ ATPase. In the later proximal tubule, the positive potential in the lumen also drives potassium reabsorption through the paracellular route.

Loop of Henle
Thin segments
Some potassium moves into the filtrate in the thin descending limb of the loop of Henle, but this is counterbalanced by movement of potassium out of the loop and into the medullary collecting ducts. The net result is some recycling of this potassium across the medullary interstitium.

Thick ascending limb
Around 30% of the filtered potassium is reabsorbed in the thick ascending limb of the loop of Henle. As in the proximal tubule, this potassium reabsorption is linked to sodium reabsorption. This is mediated by the NaK2Cl transporter, but there is also significant paracellular reabsorption, encouraged by the positive potential in the tubular lumen.

Distal tubule
The distal tubule can reabsorb more potassium and 95% of the filtered potassium is reabsorbed in a sodium-dependent fashion before the filtrate reaches the collecting ducts.

Collecting tubule and ducts
The principal cells secrete potassium whereas the intercalated cells reabsorb potassium. Generally, potassium secretion far outweighs its reabsorption in this part of the nephron. The regulation of potassium excretion occurs here and is mainly the result of changes in potassium secretion by the principal cells, rather than changes in potassium reabsorption by the intercalated cells.
- **Principal cells**. The Na^+/K^+ ATPase drives potassium secretion in principal cells by pumping potassium into the cells at the basolateral surface. The basolateral surface is not very permeable to potassium, but at the apical surface potassium ions can leave the cell through potassium channels or in co-transport with chloride. The negative potential in the tubular lumen also promotes potassium secretion. As potassium secretion into the tubule is down a concentration gradient, it can continue only if the concentration of potassium in the filtrate immediately next to the apical surface is kept low. A high flow rate carries away the secreted potassium and, *the higher the flow rate, the greater the amount of potassium that can be secreted and excreted.*
- **Intercalated cells**. The reabsorption of potassium by the intercalated cells is driven by the apical H^+/K^+ ATPase which actively pumps potassium into the cell. Potassium ions leave the cells through basolateral potassium channels and so are reabsorbed.

Medullary collecting ducts
There is some potassium reabsorption in the medullary collecting ducts, but potassium reaching the medullary interstitium is largely recycled by reabsorption into the thin descending loop of Henle.

Potassium channels in the kidney
All cell types have potassium channels and there are different types of potassium channel, even within the kidney. The **ROMK channel** is present in all nephron segments except the proximal tubule and is the key secretory channel in the principal cells of the cortical collecting ducts. The channels are generally open, and are said to be inwardly rectifying because they favor potassium flow out of the cell. They are usually around 45 kDa, with two main membrane-spanning regions.

8 Renal acid–base and buffer concepts

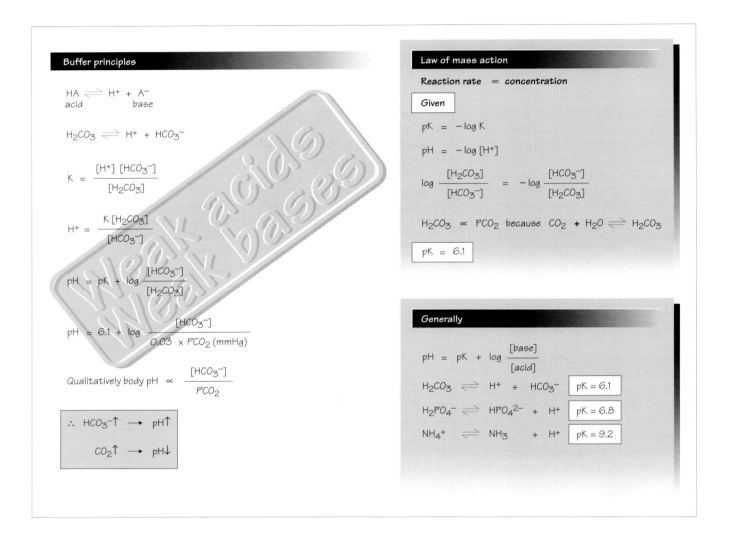

Metabolic acid production and H^+ intake must be balanced by acid excretion. Carbon dioxide produced by oxidative metabolism is excreted by the lungs, but other acids, such as sulfuric and phosphoric acids, are excreted by the kidneys. Protein metabolism produces 40–80 mmol of hydrogen ions per day, but normal extracellular pH is 7.35–7.45 or 35–45 nmol/L. As acid production is in the millimolar (10^{-3} mol/L) range, and yet plasma levels are regulated at the nanomolar (10^{-9} mol/L) level, buffers are needed to prevent huge swings in free hydrogen ion concentration. Nevertheless, buffers do not alter the body's overall H^+ load which must ultimately be excreted if the body-buffering capacity is not to be exceeded and a dangerous pH reached.

Physiologic buffers

Buffers in both blood and urine reduce the concentration of free H^+ ions. Buffers are weak acids or weak bases that are not fully dissociated. An acid can donate H^+ ions and a base can accept them. At a given H^+ concentration, a defined amount of buffer exists as acid (HA) and a defined amount as base (A^-). The ratio of buffer acid to buffer base at a given H^+ concentration is defined by the dissociation constant for an acid–base couple (pK). For a given acid–base pair, altering the ratio of the acid to the base alters the pH.

Different buffer pairs within the body are in equilibrium with each other. The main extracellular buffer is the bicarbonate system; the main intracellular buffers are sodium phosphate (Na_2HPO_4/NaH_2PO_4) and proteins. Proteins can act as bases or acids because they contain both acidic and basic amino acid side chains. As these buffer systems are in equilibrium, altering the bicarbonate system will change body pH, which resets the ratio of acid to base in the other buffers. The lungs alter the bicarbonate system by altering the carbon dioxide partial pressure ($P\text{CO}_2$) and the kidneys by altering the HCO_3^- concentration.

Acid excretion

The body can excrete acid by the urinary loss of H^+ ions associated with a buffer or by the excretion of H^+ ions as ammonium ions (NH_4^+). As hydrogen secretion into urine is inhibited below pH 4.4, this is the minimum urine pH that can be obtained. The presence of buffers in the urine allows far greater quantities of H^+ ions to be excreted above this pH than would be possible if only free H^+ ions were excreted. The major independent urinary buffer is sodium phosphate. Phosphate that is not bound to protein is freely filtered in the glomerulus and around 75% is reabsorbed. The rest is available for buffering in the urine. Nevertheless, phosphate excretion cannot be increased indefinitely and as the pK_a of phosphate is 6.8, around 90% of its buffering capacity is used up before the urinary pH drops below 5.7.

Consequently, most acid excretion occurs as a result of ammonium ion excretion.

Charge and permeability

A number of compounds such as CO_2, H_2O, and NH_3 can cross cell membranes relatively easily. However, if they are converted into their charged counterparts such as HCO_3^-, NH_4^+, H^+, OH^-, etc., these charged particles are much less able to diffuse across the cell membrane.

Carbonic anhydrase

Carbonic anhydrase catalyzes the reaction

$$OH^- + CO_2 \rightleftharpoons HCO_3^-$$

As water must first dissociate to form H^+ and OH^- for this reaction, it is usually written as

$$H_2O + CO_2 \rightleftharpoons H_2CO_3 \rightleftharpoons H^+ + HCO_3^-$$

The active site of the enzyme is a cone-shaped cavity with a zinc ion at its narrowest point. In the kidney, type II carbonic anhydrase is free in the cell cytoplasm and type IV is bound to the cell surface membrane.

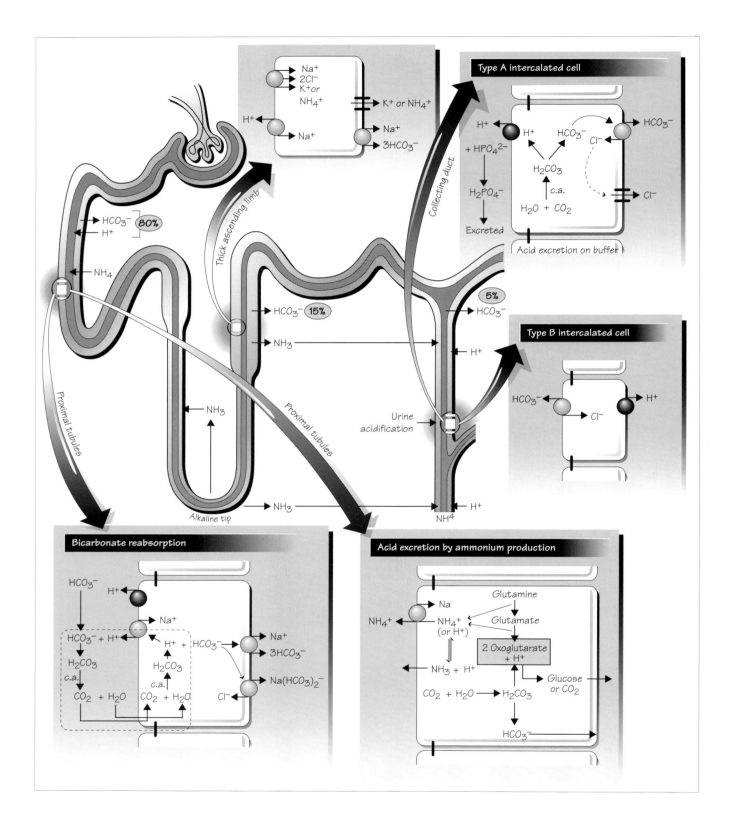

Bicarbonate reabsorption

Bicarbonate is freely filtered in the glomerulus, but most of the filtered bicarbonate is subsequently reabsorbed to maintain normal plasma bicarbonate concentration and therefore the plasma pH. Bicarbonate reabsorption depends on the secretion of H^+ ions into the lumen of the tubule. These H^+ ions are recycled by carbonic anhydrase (see Chapter 8) and there is no net acid excreted.

Hydrogen ion secretion and its effects

• When secreted H^+ ions interact with bicarbonate in the filtrate, the end result is bicarbonate reabsorption.
• However, when secreted H^+ ions interact with a urinary buffer (mainly phosphate or NH_3) the end result is the excretion of acid. When buffered acid excretion occurs, the new bicarbonate generated in the renal cells by carbonic anhydrase is added to the blood.

The secretion of H^+ ions is used to reabsorb bicarbonate early in the nephron, and it is only in the more distal nephron, when this bicarbonate reabsorption is complete, that the secreted H^+ ions interact with phosphate buffers and net acid excretion occurs. This happens because the pK_a of the bicarbonate system is 6.1, whereas that of the phosphate system is 6.8. At the initial filtrate pH of around 7.4 (similar to plasma), there is a much greater supply of bicarbonate base than of phosphate base. As bicarbonate is reabsorbed, urinary pH falls and the buffers accept H^+ ions.

Ammonia handling and acid–base balance

Tubular cells, principally those in the proximal tubule, metabolize glutamine to produce ammonia and, ultimately, glucose and bicarbonate. The bicarbonate enters the blood and the NH_4^+ ions (which effectively carry a H^+ ion) are excreted in the urine. NH_3 enters the filtrate from the tubular cells by simple diffusion or by the Na^+/H^+ exchanger, which can also transport NH_4^+. Once in the lumen, NH_3 is protonated to form NH_4^+ which cannot diffuse out of the tubules. In the thick ascending limb of the loop of Henle, NH_4^+ can be transported out of the lumen in place of K^+ on the NaK2Cl co-transporter. Also, as the tip of the loop of Henle is alkaline, NH_4^+ in the filtrate dissociates to form NH_3 and this diffuses into the interstitium. Subsequently, ammonia can diffuse back from both these sites into the thin descending limb, to be recycled in a counter-current fashion, or it can diffuse into the acidified distal tubules where it is protonated to NH_4^+ and excreted in the urine.

Tubular handling of H^+ and HCO_3^-
Proximal tubule

Of the filtered bicarbonate, 80% is reabsorbed in the proximal tubule. Most proximal tubule H^+ secretion serves this purpose and does not contribute to net acid excretion. Carbonic anhydrase in the proximal tubule cell cytoplasm and the tubular lumen facilitates the reabsorption of bicarbonate by recycling the secreted H^+ ions.

Most H^+ ions enter the filtrate via the Na^+/H^+ exchanger (NHE-3) at the apical membrane of the tubular cells. This protein is one of a family of molecules with 10–12 transmembrane regions, and is inhibited by cAMP and protein kinase A-mediated phosphorylation of its cytoplasmic tail. Na^+/H^+ exchange is linked to sodium reabsorption and is dependent ultimately on the activity of the basolateral Na^+/K^+ ATPase. The basolateral $Na^+/3HCO_3^-$ co-transporter carries most of the bicarbonate out of the cell and into the peritubular plasma. Some $Na(HCO_3)_2^-/Cl^-$ counter-transport also occurs.

Loop of Henle

A further 10–15% of filtered bicarbonate is reabsorbed in the thick ascending limb of the loop of Henle. The mechanisms responsible are similar to those in the proximal tubule and again involve carbonic anhydrase.

Distal nephron

Here, secreted H^+ ions either contribute to the reabsorption of any remaining bicarbonate or interact with urinary buffers to allow acid excretion. H^+ ions are buffered by phosphate and NH_3, which diffuses in from the medullary interstitium. Secreted H^+ ions that interact with buffers are not recycled and the new bicarbonate formed in the cell enters the blood. In the early distal tubule, Na^+/H^+ exchange still mediates most H^+ secretion but, more distally, the H^+ ATPase performs this role. The connecting tubule and cortical collecting duct contain two types of intercalated cells that are rich in carbonic anhydrase.
• **Type A** intercalated cells secrete H^+ ions. Principally this is performed by an apical H^+ ATPase, but also to a lesser extent by a H^+/K^+ ATPase similar to that in the stomach. The bicarbonate generated in the cell exits basolaterally via a HCO_3^-/Cl^- anion exchanger known as AE-1 and similar to the band-3 molecule on red blood cells.
• **Type B** intercalated cells are similar to functionally inverted type A cells with a basolateral H^+ ATPase and an apical HCO_3^-/Cl^- exchanger. Present only in the connecting tubule and cortical collecting duct, these cells secrete bicarbonate, but their role in normal acid–base homeostasis is unclear.

The principal cells play no direct role in acid–base handling, but their reabsorption of sodium generates a negative potential in the lumen, promoting H^+ secretion by type A intercalated cells.

10 Calcium, phosphate, and magnesium metabolism

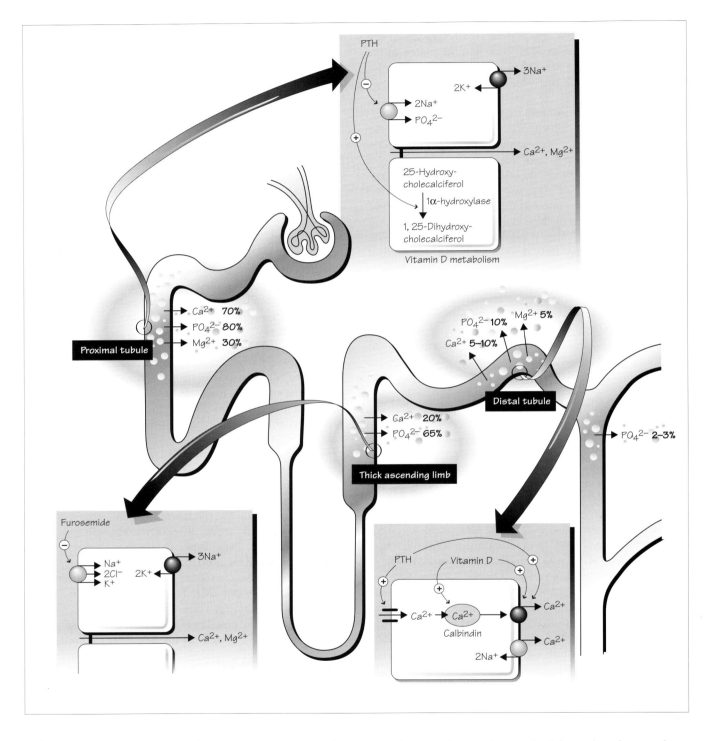

Calcium is the most prevalent divalent cation in the body, followed by magnesium; phosphate is the major divalent anion. All three occur mainly in bone. Most bone is continuously being resorbed and rebuilt at a slow rate. A more rapid bone surface exchange of calcium, phosphate, and to a lesser extent magnesium, maintains plasma levels of these ions. Plasma calcium and phosphate concentrations are close to the saturation product (calcium ion concentration times the phosphate ion concentration or $[Ca^{2+}] \times [PO_4^{2-}]$) at which calcium phosphate complexes precipitate out of solution on to the bone matrix. Plasma values of the two ions are therefore inversely related because a rise in $[Ca^{2+}]$ or $[PO_4^{3-}]$ causes some precipitation of calcium phosphate into bone with a fall in $[PO_4^{3-}]$ or $[Ca^{2+}]$ respectively.

Inside cells, calcium regulates many processes. Intracellular calcium ion concentration is kept very low; most calcium is bound to proteins or sequestered in the endoplasmic reticulum and mitochondria.

In plasma, calcium, phosphate, and magnesium can bind to protein, complex with other ions (forming calcium phosphate or magnesium phosphate), or exist as free ions. Only protein-bound ions are not filtered in the glomerulus.

Regulation of divalent ion levels is mainly by control of bone turnover and gut absorption for calcium, renal handling for magnesium, and all three mechanisms for phosphate.

Calcium

Of dietary calcium, 25–30% is absorbed by the gut, mainly in the duodenum and proximal jejunum. Absorption occurs by a transcellular process involving intracellular calcium-binding proteins called calbindins. Gut absorption is increased by vitamin D and during pregnancy. Total plasma calcium concentration is around 2.5 mmol/L, of which 45% is protein bound, 5% is complexed to other ions, and 50% (1.25 mmol/L) is free ionized Ca^{2+}.

Renal handling of calcium

In the glomerulus, calcium that is not protein bound is freely filtered and there is reabsorption along the nephron.

Of filtered calcium, 70% is reabsorbed in the proximal tubule and a further 20% in the thick ascending limb of the loop of Henle. This reabsorption is mainly passive and paracellular, and driven by sodium reabsorption. Sodium reabsorption causes water reabsorption, which raises tubular calcium concentration, causing calcium to diffuse out of the tubules. The positive lumen potential also encourages calcium to leave the tubule. The thin segments of the loop of Henle are impermeable to calcium.

A further 5–10% of filtered calcium is reabsorbed in the distal tubules and there is only minor reabsorption in the collecting ducts. Calcium reabsorption in the distal tubules is active and transcellular, and is the major target for hormonal control. As the intracellular calcium concentration must be kept low, transcellular calcium movement occurs via calcium-binding proteins, as in the gut. Calcium enters the cells through calcium channels that are activated by parathyroid hormone (PTH) and is transported across the cell by calcium-binding proteins, including the calbindins. The expression of these proteins is upregulated by vitamin D. At the basolateral surface, calcium is transported out of the cell by the Ca^{2+} ATPase and by a $3Na^+/Ca^{2+}$ exchanger. The Ca^{2+} ATPase is regulated by vitamin D and PTH.

Phosphate

About 65% of dietary phosphate is absorbed, mainly in the duodenum and jejunum by a transcellular process which is enhanced by vitamin D. Of plasma phosphate, 55% exists as free phosphate in the forms HPO_4^{2-} and $H_2PO_4^-$. These ions form a buffer pair.

Renal phosphate handling

In the glomerulus, all phosphate that is not protein bound is freely filtered and there is reabsorption along the nephron. The maximum rate of reabsorption is limited and excess filtered phosphate above a threshold level (the Tm_{P_i}) is excreted. Of filtered phosphate, 80% is reabsorbed in the proximal tubules by a transcellular process that relies on sodium reabsorption. Apical phosphate entry is by co-transport with sodium on a Na^+/PO_4^{2-} co-transporter of around 52 kDa. This transporter is inhibited by PTH. How phosphate gets out of the cell is unclear.

There is no significant phosphate transport in the loop of Henle, but the distal tubules reabsorb a further 10% of the filtered phosphate and the collecting ducts a further 2–3%. The mechanism of distal phosphate reabsorption appears to be similar to that in the proximal tubules.

Magnesium

Of the body magnesium, 54% is in bone, 45% in soft tissues, and just 1% in the extracellular fluid. In the glomerulus, magnesium that is not protein bound is freely filtered and there is reabsorption along the nephron. Only 30% is reabsorbed in the proximal tubule. The majority, 65%, is reabsorbed in the thick ascending limb by passive paracellular movement driven by the transepithelial potential. Some active magnesium reabsorption may occur because there are basolateral Mg^{2+} ATPases. A further 5% is reabsorbed in the distal tubules.

Factors influencing magnesium secretion

PTH and calcitonin increase paracellular magnesium reabsorption, possibly by influencing the permeability of the epithelial tight junctions. Both loop diuretics and thiazides increase magnesium excretion. Magnesium handling in the distal tubule and loop of Henle is directly influenced by the action of plasma magnesium ions on the Ca^{2+}/Mg^{2+} sensor on the capillary side of the tubular cells.

Drug effects on calcium excretion

Passive proximal calcium reabsorption depends on sodium reabsorption, so diuretics such as furosemide, which inhibit proximal or thick ascending loop sodium reabsorption, inhibit calcium reabsorption. In contrast, thiazides, which inhibit distal sodium reabsorption, do not inhibit active transcellular distal calcium reabsorption and can even enhance calcium reabsorption.

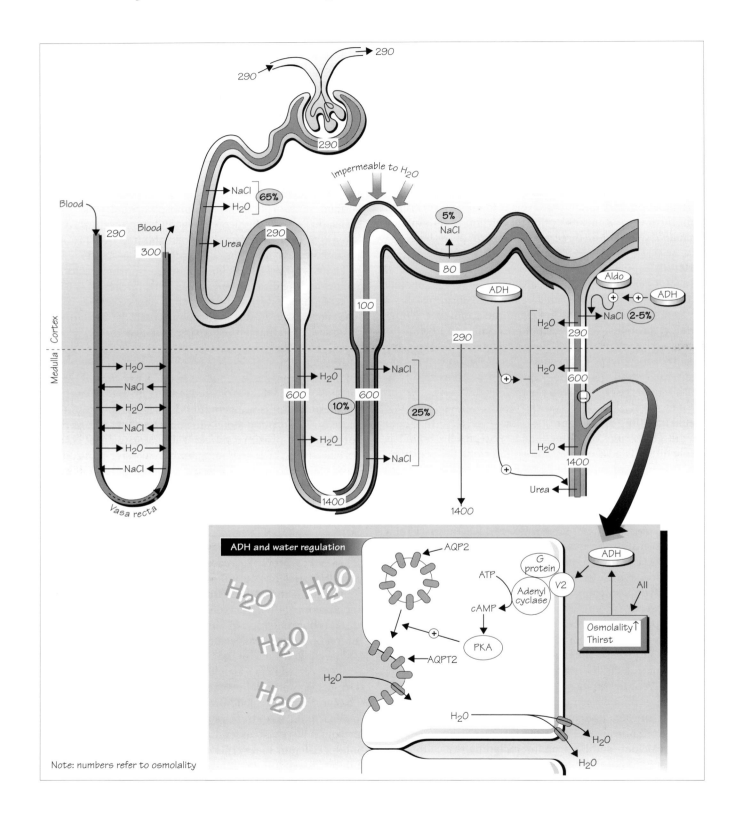

Renal handling of water

The kidney regulates body water and sodium content in parallel to maintain body volume and osmolality (normally 285–295 mosmol/kg) (see Chapter 17). The maximum urine osmolality is 1400 mosmol/kg and, as 600 mosmol of waste products must be excreted daily, the minimal daily urine volume is 600/1400 = 0.43 L.

In the glomerulus, water and ions are freely filtered. As the filtrate moves along the tubules, ions are reabsorbed and water follows by osmosis. Water reabsorption is influenced by the water permeability of the tubular epithelium and the osmotic gradient across the epithelium.

Proximal tubule

The proximal tubule is highly water permeable. As ions are reabsorbed, water follows by osmosis. This isotonic reabsorption reduces the filtrate volume, but does not alter its osmolality. Around 65% of the filtrate is reabsorbed, driven by active sodium transport.

Loop of Henle

The descending limb is permeable to water, but not ions, whereas the ascending limb (both thick and thin sections) is permeable to ions, but not water. Sodium and chloride are transported out of the thick ascending limb into the medullary interstitium. This raises the osmolality in the interstitium, which promotes water movement out of the descending limb. Within the loop, the transport of water and ions is separated with reabsorption of 25% of filtered sodium and chloride, but only 10% of filtered water. This produces a dilute urine and a hypertonic medullary interstitium. The movement of ions and water between the descending and ascending limbs creates a gradient of osmolality, which increases with depth in the medulla.

Distal tubules

The distal convoluted tubules have low water permeability and do not reabsorb water. However, reabsorption of ions further dilutes the tubular fluid.

Collecting system

The hypotonic urine passes down the collecting ducts where water permeability is controlled by antidiuretic hormone (ADH or vasopressin).
- If the permeability of the collecting ducts is low, there is no water reabsorption, but sodium chloride reabsorption continues which further dilutes the urine.
- If the permeability of the collecting ducts is high, water moves out of the hypotonic tubular fluid into the surrounding interstitium. In the cortical collecting duct, tubular fluid equilibrates with the cortical interstitium which is at plasma osmolality. In the deeper medullary collecting duct, tubular fluid then equilibrates with the high osmolality of the medullary interstitium, producing a concentrated urine.

Overall, sodium and chloride transport out of the ascending limb of the loop of Henle creates a hypertonic medullary interstitium, which drives water reabsorption from the descending limb and the medullary collecting duct. All collecting ducts pass through the medulla, so even nephrons without long loops of Henle can benefit from the hypertonic medulla.

Role of urea

Although urea is passively reabsorbed in the proximal tubule, the nephron beyond is impermeable to urea up to the inner medullary collecting duct. As water is removed along the nephron, tubular urea concentration rises. In the inner medullary collecting duct, urea is passively reabsorbed by the ADH-enhanced urea transporter 2. This reabsorbed urea accounts for half of the medullary interstitial osmolality that drives water reabsorption from the descending limb and medullary collecting duct.

Vasa recta and countercurrent exchange

If the medulla had normal blood capillaries, the interstitium would equilibrate with plasma. However, the only blood vessels supplying the medulla are the paired descending and ascending vessels called the vasa recta, which function as countercurrent exchangers. As the vessels descend into the medulla, water diffuses out and solutes into the vessels. As the vessels ascend out of the medulla, water diffuses back in and solutes out of the vessels. The result is no net change in medullary water and solute content—the medullary osmolality therefore stays high.

ADH and water regulation

ADH is a nine amino acid peptide made in the supraoptic and paraventricular nuclei of the hypothalamus. It is packaged into granules, which pass down axons to the posterior pituitary and are released by exocytosis. Osmoreceptors in the hypothalamus detect a rise in plasma osmolality above 280 mosmol/kg and trigger ADH release. Other stimuli to include ADH secretion, volume depletion, angiotensin II, hypoxia, hypercapnia, epinephrine (adrenaline), cortisol, sex steroids, pain, trauma, temperature, and psychogenic stimuli.

ADH binds V_2 receptors on collecting duct cells. This stimulates adenyl cyclase, raising cAMP levels and causing intracellular vesicles to fuse with the apical membrane. In their membrane, these vesicles contain water channels, especially the 29-kDa aquaporin protein, **AQP_2**. ADH also binds to V_1 receptors on vascular smooth muscle, causing vasoconstriction and enhancing the effect of aldosterone on sodium reabsorption in the distal tubule. AQP_1, a related protein in erythrocytes, forms hourglass-shaped water channels from membrane-spanning α helices.

12 Erythropoietin and anemia in renal disease

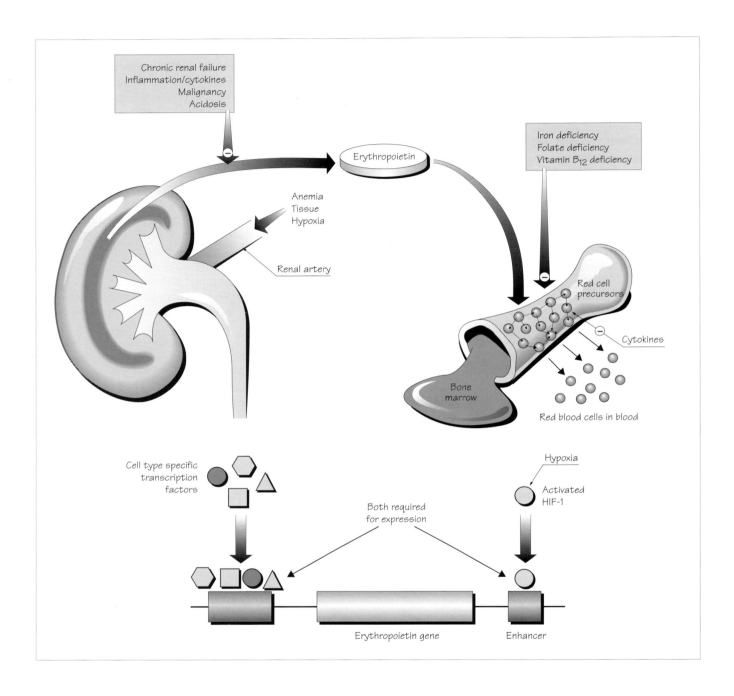

The kidney is the main source of erythropoietin, the hemopoietic growth factor that promotes red blood cell formation. Erythropoietin increases reticulocyte production and early release of reticulocytes from the bone marrow. In chronic renal failure, erythropoietin production is inadequate and there is usually anemia.

Mature erythropoietin is a heavily glycosylated protein consisting of 165 amino acids. It interacts with the erythropoietin receptor, a protein of 508 amino acids, which is homologous to other growth factor receptors. Binding of erythropoietin to its receptor results in receptor internalization, and subsequent signaling events include tyrosine phosphorylation and calcium entry. The receptor is expressed on early erythroid progenitors and the level of expression increases during red cell development. Withdrawal of erythropoietin from these precursor cells causes apoptotic cell death.

Erythropoietin production

The major site of erythropoietin production in the adult is the kidney. A small amount is also produced by the liver in some hepatocytes and in fibroblastoid Ito cells; the liver is the major site of production in the fetus and neonate. In the kidney, erythropoietin is made in type I fibroblastoid cells in the peritubular interstitium of the cortex and outer medulla. There is normally a low basal level of erythropoietin production by the kidney, but this is enhanced by anemia or a fall in arterial Po_2, situations that both cause tissue hypoxia. Hypoxia initially stimulates erythropoietin mRNA synthesis in cells in the deep cortex, but, as hypoxia progresses, cells in more superficial sites also produce erythropoietin. This distribution reflects advancing hypoxia as there is a gradient of hypoxia from the cortex to the inner medulla because the medulla receives all its blood supply from the vasa recta.

Low erythropoietin levels in response to anemia are found in chronic renal failure, inflammatory disease, malignancy, acidosis, and starvation, or with the use of angiotensin-converting enzyme inhibitors. Acidosis reduces the oxygen affinity of hemoglobin, which can promote tissue oxygenation and so reduce the stimulus to erythropoietin production. In inflammatory disease, cytokines such as tumor necrosis factor α reduce erythropoietin production and cytokines such as interferon-β suppress the erythropoietic response to erythropoietin.

Hypoxic stimulation of erythropoietin production

The exact mechanism of oxygen sensing is unclear. Hypoxia in some way activates or induces the transcription factor HIF-1 (hypoxia inducible factor). This promotes the expression of the erythropoietin gene by binding to an enhancer sequence downstream of the erythropoietin gene and promoting erythropoietin transcription. HIF-1 also acts in many different cell types to activate other genes relevant to hypoxia, such as the glycolytic enzymes. However, sequences upstream of the erythropoietin gene provide tissue-specific regulation by only allowing erythropoietin expression when other cell type-specific transcription factors are bound.

Erythropoietin and chronic renal failure

Anemia is common in chronic renal disease, but most patients do not have a raised erythropoietin level. Chronic renal disease often causes interstitial changes and the type I erythropoietin-producing cells become more myofibroblastoid with less potential for erythropoietin production. Although there may be some destruction of these erythropoietin-producing cells, the main problem is a failure of the cells to produce enough erythropoietin in response to the anemia. An exception is polycystic kidney disease where erythropoietin production is often preserved or even elevated and erythropoietin production has been demonstrated in cyst wall cells.

Other factors in chronic renal disease, such as reduced red cell survival, can contribute to the anemia which is characteristically normocytic/normochromic. However, it is always important to exclude iron deficiency resulting from poor intake or blood loss and to exclude folate deficiency or less commonly vitamin B_{12} deficiency. The serum ferritin level should be measured to exclude iron deficiency, but can be spuriously elevated if there is inflammation. Aluminum toxicity can cause a microcytic anemia like that of iron deficiency, and can be a problem in patients who have used aluminum-containing phosphate-binding agents.

Erythropoietin therapy

Renal transplantation restores normal erythropoietin production, although continued erythropoietin production from the native kidneys can cause polycythemia. Generally, peritoneal dialysis is associated with less anemia than hemodialysis, but, in both cases, erythropoietin is given to maintain a normal hemoglobin level.

Subcutaneous administration gives a more sustained rise in erythropoietin level than intravenous administration and is usually given three times weekly. Erythropoietin can cause hypertension or polycythemia, so the blood count and blood pressure are checked every 2 weeks. The dose is adjusted upwards if there is no response by 4 weeks. When the target hemoglobin is reached, it may be possible to reduce the dose to twice a week. It is important that sufficient iron is available during erythropoietin therapy — ferritin, transferrin saturation and the appearance of hypochromic cells on the blood film are useful guides to iron levels. A good response to therapy is first indicated by a rise in the reticulocyte count.

The major complications are polycythemia, hypertension, and thrombosis of vascular access sites used for dialysis. Resistance to erythropoietin therapy often reflects iron deficiency, inflammation, or malignancy. Severe hyperparathyroidism can blunt the response to erythropoietin, possibly because of bone marrow fibrosis.

Acute renal failure

In acute renal failure, anemia usually represents blood loss or hemolysis. Although erythropoietin levels often fail to rise appropriately, the patients are usually unwell, often with ongoing sepsis or inflammation which render erythropoietin ineffective.

13 Renal vascular biology

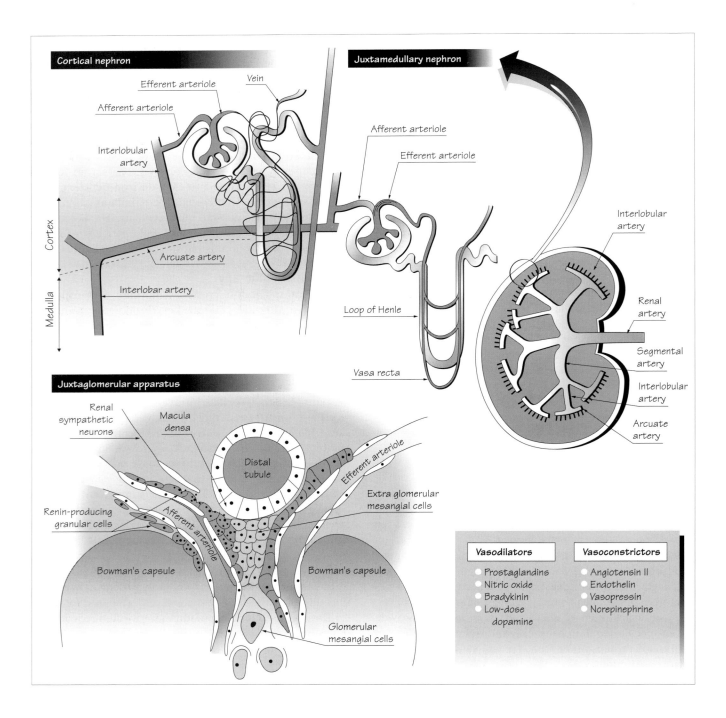

Each kidney is supplied by a renal artery arising from the aorta. Within the kidney, the renal artery divides into two or three segmental arteries, which further subdivide into interlobar arteries and then into arcuate arteries. The arcuate arteries curve parallel to the outer surface of the kidney, giving rise to the interlobular arteries, which ascend through the cortex and give off the afferent arterioles that supply the glomerular capillary bed. Beyond the glomeruli, the capillaries regroup as efferent arterioles. In the outer cortex, these give rise to peritubular capillaries which surround the tubules. Efferent arterioles arising from the juxtamedullary nephrons descend into the medulla and give rise to the vasa recta, which descend and re-ascend in close proximity to the loops of Henle. Blood leaves the kidney in veins that travel with the corresponding arteries and join to form a single renal vein, which enters the inferior vena cava.

Renal blood flow

Together the kidneys receive a renal blood flow (RBF) of 1000 mL/min which is 20% of the cardiac output. The normal hematocrit is 0.45, so red cells account for 45% of RBF and the renal plasma flow (RPF) is 550 mL/min. The glomerular filtration rate (GFR) is about 120 mL/min, so the filtration fraction (FF = GFR/RPF), which is the proportion of plasma that is filtered, is around 20%. Renal vascular resistance arises mainly from the afferent and efferent arterioles. High pressure in the glomerular capillaries forces filtrate through the filtration barrier. This pressure is reduced by afferent arteriolar constriction and increased by efferent arteriolar constriction.

Measuring renal blood and plasma flow

The amount of a substance removed from plasma by the kidneys in 1 min (arterial–venous concentration × RPF) equals the amount appearing in the urine in 1 min (urine flow/min × urine concentration). If arterial, venous, and urinary concentration and urine flow are measured, RPF can be calculated. This can be done after an injection of *p*-aminohippuric acid (PAH) which is fully removed after a single pass through the kidney. RBF can be calculated from the RPF if the hemotocrit is known:

$$RBF = RPF/(1 - Hematocrit)$$

^{99m}Tc-labeled DTPA (diethylenetriaminepenta-acetic acid) and MAG$_3$ (mercaptoacetyl-triglycine) are both removed by the kidney so, in clinical practice, they can be detected by a gamma camera to estimate RBF.

Regulation of renal blood flow

Autoregulation
• *Myogenic reflex.* A rise in pressure stretches the blood vessel, causing reflex vasoconstriction which reduces flow.
• *Tubuloglomerular feedback.* If glomerular pressure is increased, GFR and therefore tubular flow rate also increase. This reduces the time available for sodium and chloride reabsorption in the ascending loop of Henle. The higher tubular sodium and chloride concentrations detected by the macula densa cause the juxtaglomerular apparatus (JGA) to release substances such as adenosine. This causes afferent arteriolar vasoconstriction which reduces GFR.

Renin–angiotensin II system
The JGA releases renin in response to a drop in afferent arteriolar pressure, a fall in tubular flow rate, or a rise in tubular sodium and chloride concentration at the macula densa. Other stimuli include sympathetic nerve stimulation of β$_1$-adrenergic receptors on granular cells and a fall in angiotensin II (AII) levels. Renin promotes production of AII which acts via AII receptors to vasoconstrict afferent and efferent arterioles. The dominant effect is on efferent arteriolar constriction, so the GFR is increased.

Prostaglandins
Many peripheral vasoconstrictors especially AII, ADH, endothelin, and norepinephrine (noradrenaline) stimulate the renal production of vasodilating prostaglandins such as PGE$_2$ and PGI$_2$ (prostacyclin). This protects the kidney from severe vasoconstriction.

Vasoactive peptides
• *Bradykinin* is a peptide of nine amino acids released from a precursor kallidin by the enzyme kallikrein in the distal tubule and glomerulus. It acts on B$_1$- and B$_2$-receptors, promoting prostaglandin synthesis and vasodilation.
• *Atrial natriuretic peptide* (ANP) is released from cardiac cells and can produce systemic vasodilation.
• *Endothelin* is a peptide of 21 amino acids made in renal vascular endothelial cells and tubules. It is a potent vasoconstrictor. It acts via the phosphoinositide messenger system and promotes calcium entry into cells. In the periphery, endothelin acts mainly on ET$_A$-receptors; in the kidney, it acts mainly on ET$_B$-receptors.
• *Vasopressin (ADH)* promotes vasoconstriction via V$_1$-receptors and antidiuretic action via V$_2$-receptors.

Other regulatory pathways
• *Renal nerves* contain sympathetic neurons which release norepinephrine (noradrenaline). Like circulating epinephrine (adrenaline), this acts via G-protein-linked α$_1$-receptors, causing constriction of afferent and efferent arterioles. Renin release is also promoted.
• *Dopamine* is used clinically to promote renal blood flow. At low concentrations (1–3 µg/kg per min), it has a vasodilatory effect through DA$_1$-receptors acting via cAMP. At higher concentrations, dopamine causes renal vasoconstriction via α$_1$-receptors and through β$_1$-receptor-mediated renin release.
• *Nitric oxide (NO)* is a potent vasodilator that acts via cGMP and regulates renal vascular smooth muscle tone. It is synthesized from L-arginine by NO synthases in the macula densa, endothelium, and mesangial cells. It has a short half-life and is upregulated in response to mechanical sheer stress.
• *Adenosine* produces vasoconstriction via A$_1$-receptors and vasodilation via A$_2$-receptors.

14 Drug and organic molecule handling by the kidney

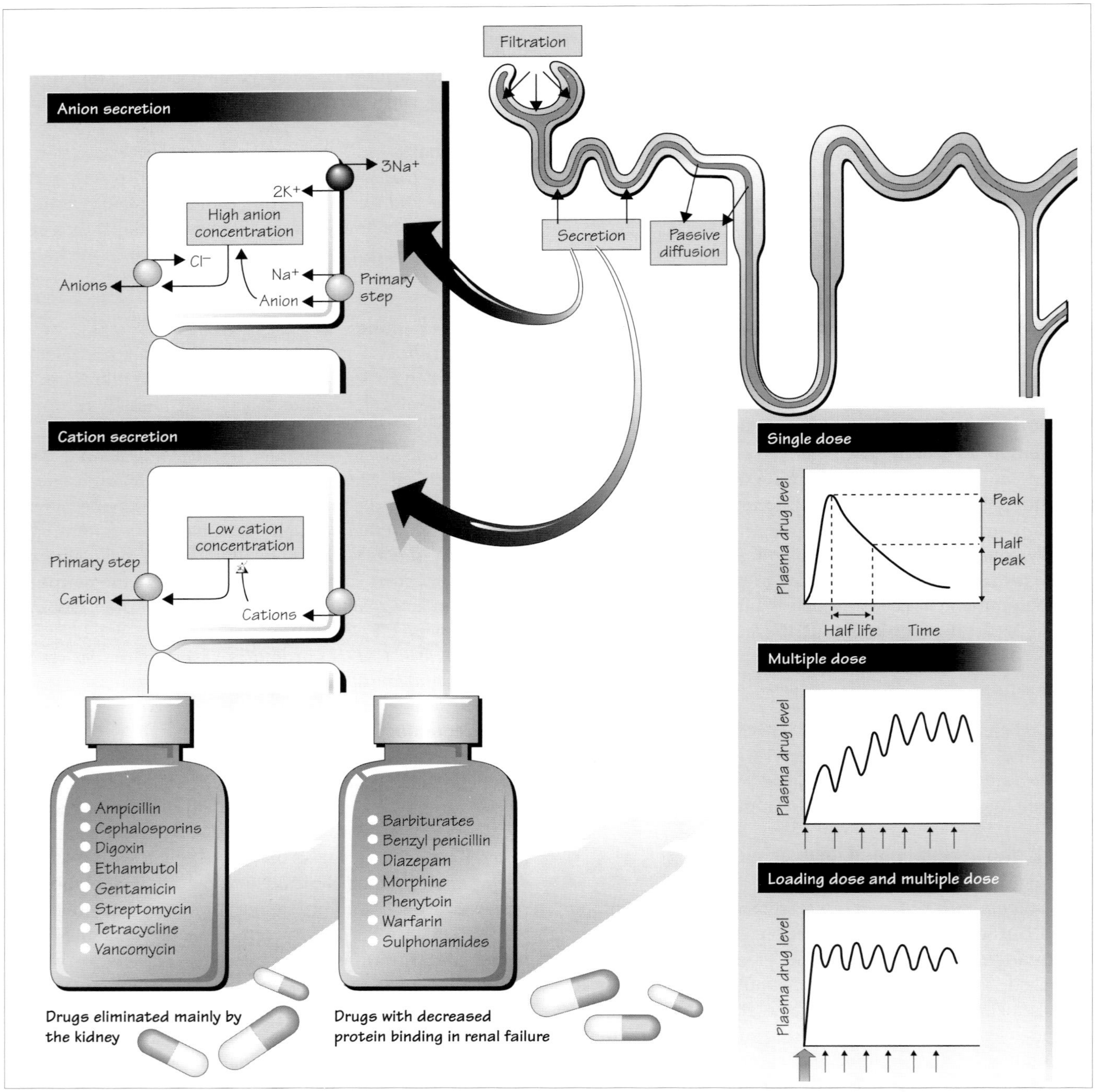

Filtration

Anion secretion

$3Na^+$
$2K^+$
High anion concentration
Cl^-
Anions
Na^+
Anion
Primary step

Secretion
Passive diffusion

Cation secretion

Low cation concentration
Primary step
Cation
Cations

Single dose

Plasma drug level

Peak
Half peak

Half life   Time

Multiple dose

Plasma drug level

Loading dose and multiple dose

Plasma drug level

Ampicillin
Cephalosporins
Digoxin
Ethambutol
Gentamicin
Streptomycin
Tetracycline
Vancomycin

Barbiturates
Benzyl penicillin
Diazepam
Morphine
Phenytoin
Warfarin
Sulphonamides

Drugs eliminated mainly by the kidney

Drugs with decreased protein binding in renal failure

Many drugs are excreted by the kidney, and can accumulate to toxic levels if there is renal impairment.

Overview of drug kinetics

Unless a drug is injected intravenously, it must be absorbed from its site of administration (usually the gut, skin, or muscle) into the blood and travel to its site of action. Most oral drugs are absorbed in the small bowel. Some drugs undergo 'first-pass metabolism' in which they are metabolized or inactivated in the liver, or less commonly in the gut or lung, before they reach the systemic circulation. Once absorbed, a drug equilibrates throughout its volume of distribution, which may include only specific tissues.

Plasma proteins bind many drugs; albumin binds acidic drugs whereas α_1-acid glycoprotein binds basic drugs. Drugs bound strongly to plasma proteins tend to stay in the circulation. If protein binding is low, the distribution depends on lipid solubility. Water-soluble drugs stay in the extracellular fluid, but lipid-soluble drugs can enter cells and can even be concentrated in adipose tissue.

Drugs can be metabolized, especially in the liver, and the activity of the metabolites may differ from that of the original drug. Phase I reactions cause oxidation, reduction, or hydrolysis of the drug and involve cytochrome P450 mixed function oxidases. Phase II interactions add groups such as glucuronides or sulfates on to phase I products to increase their water solubility. These metabolites may be excreted from the liver in bile or by the kidney.

Renal drug handling

Filtration
Drugs bound to plasma proteins are not filtered because the proteins are not filtered. Filtration of drugs that are not protein bound depends on their size and charge.

Tubular secretion
Organic anion and cation transporters in the proximal tubule can transport drugs and are saturable. Tubular reabsorption of drugs is of little importance.

Anions are co-transported with sodium across the basolateral cell surface. This process is fueled by the sodium gradient established by the Na^+/K^+ ATPase. The anions then travel down their concentration gradient and enter the tubular lumen in exchange for another anion such as Cl^-.

Cations are transported across the apical membrane. This promotes basolateral cation entry along a concentration gradient, probably via a passive transporter. Cation transport may be fueled by both sodium and proton gradients across the apical membrane.

Cationic drugs do not accumulate in tubular cells because they are transported out of the cell at the apical membrane. However, anionic drugs can accumulate to toxic level because they are transported into the cell at the basolateral membrane. Probenecid inhibits the excretion of pencillins by the anion transporter and has been used to increase penicillin levels in plasma.

Passive diffusion
Lipid-soluble drugs diffuse through cell membranes and across tubular cells. As the urine is concentrated along the nephron, urine drug concentrations increase and lipid-soluble drugs diffuse back into the blood. Water-soluble drugs cannot cross cell membranes and so stay in the urine and are more efficiently excreted by the kidney.

Effect of urine pH
The pH of urine affects whether or not an organic acid or base is protonated and therefore charged. A charge favors water solubility and therefore renal excretion.

Prescribing renally excreted drugs
Renal drug excretion displays first-order kinetics. This means that the rate of drug removal is proportional to the plasma drug concentration. After a single dose, the plasma level rises, peaks, and falls. The half-life is the time taken for the peak level to halve. During steady dosing, it takes around four half-lives to reach a steady state. Administration of a dose equal to the amount of drug in the body at steady state bypasses this delay. A maintenance dose can then be half the loading dose given once every half-life. The volume of distribution of a drug is calculated by dividing the amount of a drug administered by the plasma concentration. It is the hypothetical volume of plasma that the drug would have to equilibrate into to produce the measured plasma level. Steady-state levels are raised by an increase in half-life, a reduction in the volume of distribution, higher doses, more frequent doses, and greater absorption of the drug.

Prescribing in renal impairment
Renal impairment reduces glomerular filtration and tubular secretion of drugs. It usually affects drug dosing if non-renal elimination is less than 50% of the total elimination. To avoid toxicity, either the dose or the dosing interval is reduced and when necessary drug levels are monitored.

Most polypeptide hormones, including insulin and parathyroid hormone, are metabolized by the kidney and their clearance is reduced in renal impairment. In chronic renal disease, protein binding of acidic drugs (such as phenytoin and theophylline) is reduced because uremic toxins compete for drug-binding sites on albumin. In contrast, protein binding of basic drugs is increased in uremic patients because levels of α_1-acid glycoprotein are elevated.

Dialysis
Water-soluble drugs are better removed by dialysis than lipid-soluble drugs. Heavily protein-bound drugs are poorly removed. A drug such as digoxin, with a very large volume of distribution, has a low plasma concentration and is, therefore, poorly removed. If a drug is mainly eliminated by dialysis, it is usual just to give a dose after each dialysis. Hemofiltration can remove larger molecules than hemodialysis because the membrane pore size is larger in hemofiltration than in hemodialysis. Peritoneal dialysis is relatively inefficient at clearing drugs.

15 Renal pharmacology: diuretics

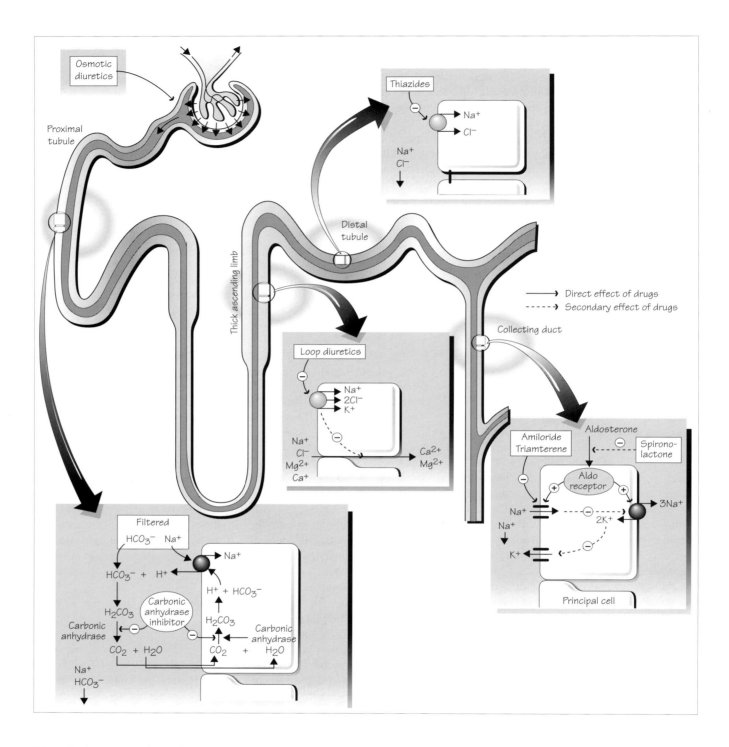

Diuretics increase urine volume. Their action increases the amount of osmotically active substances (usually sodium and chloride ions) in the tubules. This opposes water reabsorption and increases urine volume.

Loop diuretics

Loop diuretics are strong diuretics and include furosemide, bumetanide, and ethacrynic acid. They are highly plasma bound, but are secreted into the tubule by the organic anion transporter. They bind the NaK2Cl co-transporter in the thick ascending limb of the loop of Henle. This binding inhibits sodium, potassium and chloride reabsorption, causing diuresis with loss of these electrolytes. The transcellular voltage difference falls and paracellular calcium and magnesium reabsorption are also reduced.

Salt reabsorption in the ascending limb normally concentrates the medullary interstitium. By blocking this process, loop diuretics can reduce the ability of the kidney to concentrate urine (see Chapter 11). Increased sodium delivery to the principal cells in the collecting duct increases potassium secretion in return for sodium reabsorption.

Clinical aspects

The relationship between furosemide dose and effect is approximately logarithmic and a small increase in effect requires a large increase in dose. Usually a doubling is required. During long-term use, distal tubule hypertrophy can reduce the efficacy of loop diuretics and additional inhibition of distal tubule sodium reabsorption by thiazides (especially metolazone) can be useful. This has been termed 'serial nephron blockade'.

In edema states, gut edema impairs absorption of oral furosemide, so intravenous administration can be more effective. Acute intravenous infusion also promotes venodilation, possibly by triggering renal prostaglandin production. Experimentally, loop diuretics reduce energy consumption, helping tubular cells to survive ischemia. However, they do not improve the outcome from renal ischemia in humans.

Adverse effects include sodium, potassium, magnesium, and water depletion. In the long term, plasma and tissue urate levels can rise triggering gout.

Thiazides: the distal tubular diuretics

Thiazides are generally weak diuretics and are secreted into the proximal tubule. They reversibly inhibit the apical NaCl co-transporter in the early distal tubule by binding to the chloride-binding site. More sodium is delivered to the principal cells of the collecting duct. Some of this excess sodium is exchanged for potassium, causing hypokalemia. Calcium reabsorption is increased, possibly because of increased basolateral Na^+/Ca^{2+} exchange, and thiazides can be used to treat hypercalciuria. Thiazides are also used to treat hypertension because they decrease peripheral resistance, but the mechanism of this action is not clear.

Adverse effects include sodium, potassium, chloride, and magnesium depletion. Cholesterol and urate levels can rise.

Potassium-sparing collecting duct diuretics

Amiloride and *triamterene* are mainly used to reduce potassium loss caused by loop diuretics. In the principal cells of the cortical collecting duct, sodium entry from the lumen via the epithelial sodium channel (ENaC) is associated with apical potassium exit. Sodium reabsorption is therefore linked to potassium secretion and both depend on the activity of the basolateral Na^+/K^+ ATPase. Amiloride competes with sodium for a site in the ENaC channel and thus blocks sodium reabsorption and potassium secretion. Triamterene has a similar action.

Aldosterone promotes sodium reabsorption and potassium secretion by increasing transcription of the ENaC channel and the Na^+/K^+ ATPase. *Spironolactone* blocks aldosterone receptors (type 1 mineralocorticoid receptors), so reducing sodium reabsorption and potassium secretion.

Adverse effects of potassium-sparing diuretics include hyperkalemia and, in the case of spironolactone, an antiandrogenic effect that can cause gynecomastia. The antibiotics pentamidine and trimethoprim can cause hyperkalemia by an amiloride-like action.

Carbonic anhydrase inhibitors

Carbonic anhydrase inhibitors block the reaction of carbon dioxide and water and so prevent Na^+/H^+ exchange and bicarbonate reabsorption (see Chapters 8 & 9). The increased bicarbonate levels in the filtrate oppose water reabsorption. Proximal tubule sodium reabsorption is also reduced because it is partly dependent on bicarbonate reabsorption.

Osmotic diuretics

Osmotic diuretics, such as mannitol or glycerol, are filtered in the glomerulus and then not reabsorbed. As the filtrate passes along the nephron, water is reabsorbed and the concentration of the osmotic diuretic rises until its osmotic effect opposes further reabsorption of water. Sodium is then reabsorbed without water. Eventually, sodium reabsorption is also inhibited because the sodium gradient between filtrate and plasma increases to the point at which sodium leaks back into the lumen.

Mannitol, an osmotic diuretic, draws water from cells osmotically and is used to dehydrate brain cells in cerebral edema. It enhances renal blood flow by increasing extracellular and intravascular volume and reducing red cell volume and blood viscosity. Enhanced blood flow can reduce the medullary interstitial osmolality, reducing the urinary-concentrating capacity. Mannitol infusion is sometimes given to prevent acute renal failure in high-risk settings. Its benefit is controversial and excess infusion can cause volume overload if renal function is impaired.

Glucose is filtered in the glomerulus. A high plasma glucose level causes a high filtrate glucose level, which can exceed the tubular capacity for its reabsorption. Glucose then acts as an osmotic diuretic causing volume depletion during diabetic hyperglycemia. High levels of *urea* from protein metabolism can also promote an osmotic diuresis in a functioning kidney.

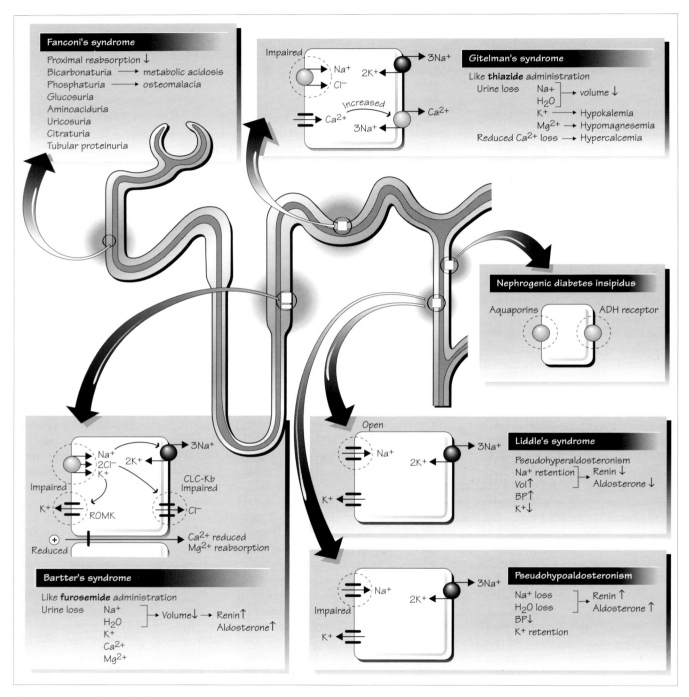

Genetic mutations of channels and transporters

Genetic mutations in the channels involved in sodium, potassium, and chloride handling can produce very similar effects to the diuretic drugs that act on the same channels.

The NaK2Cl co-transporter

Mutations that impair the activity of the NaK2Cl co-transporter in the thick ascending limb of the loop of Henle cause *Bartter's syndrome*. This condition is characterized by excessive urinary sodium, potassium, and water loss—effects similar to those of furosemide, the diuretic that blocks this channel. The resulting hypokalemia promotes enhanced acid secretion and metabolic alkalosis (see Chapter 25). As the mutant protein cannot transport ions, the transepithelial potential difference falls and the fluid in the tubular lumen loses its positive charge. This reduces calcium reabsorption and causes hypercalciuria, which can predispose to renal stone formation. Renin and aldosterone levels are high to conserve sodium because of volume depletion.

The ROMK and CLC-Kb channels

Bartter's syndrome can also result from mutations in the apical ROMK potassium channel or the basolateral CLC-Kb chloride channel in the thick ascending limb of the loop of Henle. Defects in the potassium or chloride channels block the efficient exit of these ions from the cell, and this inhibits the passive entry of sodium, potassium, and chloride into the cell via the NaK2Cl transporter.

The sodium/chloride co-transporters

Mutations in the genes encoding the sodium/chloride co-transporter in the distal tubule produces *Gitelman's syndrome*. This disorder produces effects similar to those seen with the thiazide diuretics: there is excess loss of sodium, potassium, and magnesium in the urine. The excess urinary potassium loss is the result of enhanced tubular flow which increases potassium secretion in the cortical collecting duct (see Chapter 7). Hypocalciuria occurs because the inhibition of apical sodium entry into the cell allows more basolateral sodium/calcium exchange, and therefore more apical calcium entry and greater calcium reabsorption.

The ENaC channels

Different mutations in the ENaC sodium channel in the collecting ducts can switch the channel on or off.

Activating mutations—pseudohyperaldosteronism

These mutations are dominant and leave the ENaC channel open in an unregulated fashion, which causes excess sodium retention, resulting in volume expansion and hypertension and suppressing renin and aldosterone levels. These features constitute *Liddle's syndrome*. Amiloride can be helpful because it blocks the channel. Liddle's syndrome causes pseudohyperaldosteronism by mimicking the effects of aldosterone and causing sodium retention and potassium loss.

Inactivating mutations—pseudohypoaldosteronism

In the ENaC sodium channel, these mutations are recessive and cause excessive sodium loss and potassium retention. These effects promote high renin and high aldosterone levels. The aldosterone cannot exert its effect because of the reduced function of the ENaC channel, with resulting pseudohypoaldosteronism. The condition therefore mimics aldosterone deficiency.

Chloride channels and renal stone formation

Mutations in the voltage-gated chloride channels CLC-5 and CLC-Kb cause hypercalciuric nephrolithiasis. CLC-Kb mutations are discussed above. Mutations in CLC-5 cause Dent's disease, X-linked recessive hypophosphatemic rickets, and low-molecular-weight proteinuria with hypercalciuria and nephrocalcinosis. These diseases are basically similar and differ mainly in severity. The main features are reduced calcium reabsorption and hypercalciuria, causing renal stone formation, nephrocalcinosis, and in some cases renal failure.

Water channels

Nephrogenic diabetes insipidus can result from defects in the aquaporins or the V_2 ADH receptors in the collecting duct (see Chapter 18).

Fanconi's syndrome

There are many inherited and acquired forms of Fanconi's syndrome and only part of the full spectrum of proximal tubular disorders may be present. The major components of Fanconi's syndrome are proximal renal tubular acidosis (caused by reduced bicarbonate reabsorption), glucosuria, aminoaciduria, uricosuria (urinary urate loss) with hypouricemia, citraturia, and phosphate loss with hypophosphatemia and osteomalacia or rickets. There may also be tubular proteinuria as a result of a failure of tubular reabsorption of small proteins and hypokalemia resulting from enhanced distal sodium delivery, which promotes distal potassium secretion. The osmotic load may cause an osmotic diuresis and polyuria.

The syndrome can result from any cause of proximal tubular damage. Causes include vitamin D-dependent rickets caused by defects in the vitamin D_3 receptor or in the renal 1α-hydroxylase enzyme involved in vitamin D synthesis. Metabolic defects in sugar and carbohydrate metabolism, and conditions such as Wilson's disease with abnormal copper deposition, can also cause proximal tubular defects. Cystinosis is a rare condition in which there is excess cystine in the blood and cystine deposition can cause proximal tubular damage.

Carbonic anhydrase II deficiency (Guibaud–Vainsel syndrome) results in both proximal and distal **renal tubular acidosis** because bicarbonate reabsorption is impaired throughout the nephron. Glucose is reabsorbed by co-transport with sodium in the proximal tubule and defects in the sodium/glucose transporter-2 (SGLT-2) result in **glucosuria**. Defects in amino acid reabsorption in the proximal tubule can cause **aminoacidurias**. The most common is cystinuria which results in cystine stone formation (see Chapter 47).

Regulation of body sodium and body water

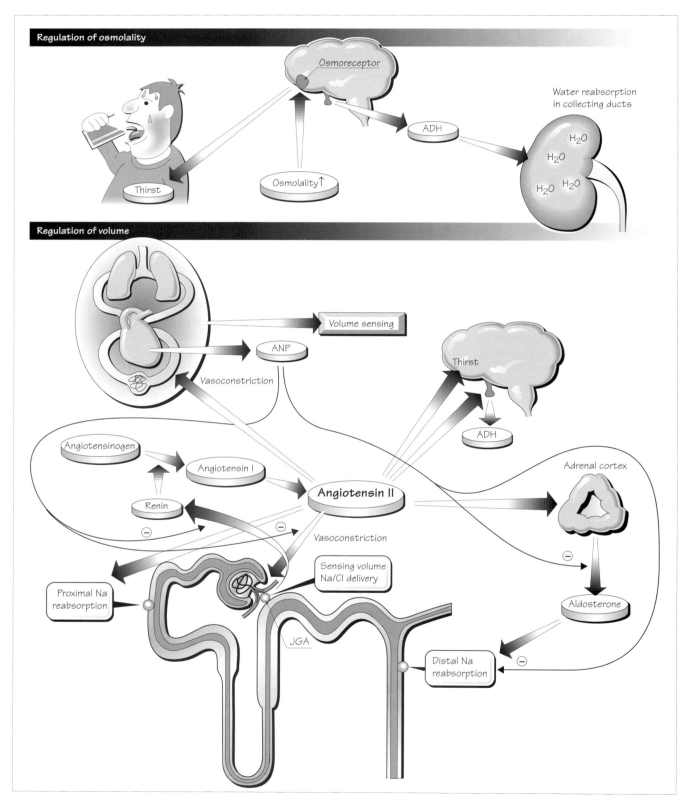

Total body volume reflects total body water content. The body senses osmolality and body volume, and regulates them by altering water and sodium content, respectively. Water can be moved only by osmosis and, as the major osmotically active extracellular ions are sodium salts, sodium and water regulation are tightly linked. The body directly controls the osmolality and volume of the intravascular extracellular fluid and this influences the osmolality and volumes of the other compartments.

Body water exists in the extracellular and intracellular compartments. The extracellular compartment consists of the intravascular and extravascular spaces, which are in approximate equilibrium. Sodium salts account for around 280 of the total 290 mosmol/kg H_2O in the extracellular fluid. As sodium is actively pumped out of cells, sodium salts account for only 40 of the total 290 mosmol/kg H_2O in the intracellular fluid.

Regulation of osmolality

Unless there is a massive volume change, such as an acute bleed, osmolality is usually maintained at the expense of volume changes. All body compartments are in approximate osmotic equilibrium and there is only one set of osmoreceptors in the anterior hypothalamus, near the supraoptic nuclei. *The osmoreceptors control water intake by altering thirst and renal water excretion by altering ADH release.*

Changes in sodium concentration influence osmolality. For example, salt ingestion raises plasma osmolality, provoking thirst and reducing renal water excretion. This increases body volume and reduces salt concentration and osmolality, but it does not alter the amount of salt present. Thus, osmoregulation controls plasma sodium concentration by altering the water balance, but it does not control body sodium content.

Regulation of volume

If the body sodium content is altered, the osmoregulatory system adjusts water balance and therefore the body volume to maintain normal osmolality. Body volume can be controlled by altering body sodium content. The kidney controls sodium excretion and therefore body volume. Body volume sensing is complex and there are multiple volume receptors. This input is integrated by the nervous system to produce a coordinated neural and endocrine response that regulates renal sodium excretion.

Sensing body volume

Baroreceptors respond to vascular stretch. High-pressure arterial stretch receptors can detect low perfusion pressure, usually when the intravascular volume is too low. Low-pressure venous stretch receptors can detect whether the intravascular volume is too high. There are many receptors that detect circulatory pressure, including atrial stretch receptors, the carotid baroreceptors, the juxtaglomerular apparatus and various tissue mechanoreceptors. Many of these receptors have neural links to the hypothalamus and medulla.

Control of renal sodium excretion

Angiotensin II binds to AT1-receptors in the proximal tubule, activating the phosphoinositol secondary messenger system. This promotes apical Na^+/H^+ exchange and therefore sodium reabsorption. Angiotensin II also causes thirst and stimulates aldosterone production, ADH release, and renal and systemic vasoconstriction. Renin is released when the total body sodium falls. The stimulus is a fall in circulatory volume, which increases renal sympathetic nerve activity (mediated by β-adrenergic receptors), reduces afferent arteriolar tension, and reduces sodium chloride delivery to the macula densa.

Aldosterone diffuses into the principal cells of the collecting duct and binds to type 1 steroid receptors in the cytosol. This complex then migrates into the nucleus, promoting transcription of new apical sodium channels and basolateral Na^+/K^+ ATPases. These changes increase sodium reabsorption. Aldosterone is mainly regulated by the renin–angiotensin II system.

Atrial natriuretic peptide is stored in atrial cells as a propeptide which is cleaved and released on atrial distention. It is also produced in collecting duct cells. It binds to ANP-A-receptors on collecting duct cells and acts via cGMP to inactivate apical sodium channels, so reducing sodium reabsorption. It also inhibits aldosterone release and renin production and increases the glomerular filtration rate by dilating afferent arterioles.

Vasopressin (ADH) enhances water reabsorption in the collecting ducts. It also increases sodium reabsorption in the collecting duct by a synergistic effect with that of aldosterone.

Prostaglandins produced in the medulla, especially PGE_2, enhance sodium and water excretion and are vasodilators.

Dopamine is secreted in the proximal tubule and reduces sodium reabsorption by inhibiting Na^+/H^+ exchange. This effect is mediated by DA_1-receptors which activate adenyl cyclase; *it is opposite to that of angiotensin II and α-adrenergic agonists.* Dopamine is also a vasodilator.

α-Adrenergic agonists act via G proteins to enhance Na^+/H^+ exchange and increase sodium reabsorption in the proximal tubule.

Extracellular fluid volume directly influences sodium excretion. Proximal tubule sodium and chloride reabsorption requires the ultimate removal of these ions from the lateral intracellular spaces. If the extracellular fluid volume is increased, capillary hydrostatic pressure rises and plasma proteins are diluted, reducing the capillary osmotic pressure. These changes reduce salt and water uptake from the interspace, promoting sodium and water excretion and thus reducing the extracellular fluid volume.

18 Disorders of sodium and water metabolism

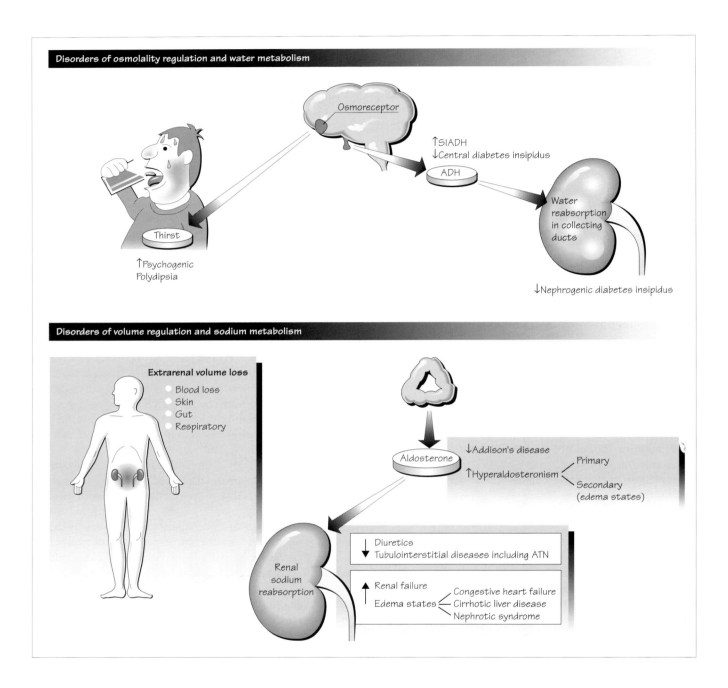

Disorders of osmolality regulation and water metabolism

Osmoreceptor

↑SIADH
↓Central diabetes insipidus

ADH

Water reabsorption in collecting ducts

Thirst

↑Psychogenic Polydipsia

↓Nephrogenic diabetes insipidus

Disorders of volume regulation and sodium metabolism

Extrarenal volume loss
- Blood loss
- Skin
- Gut
- Respiratory

Aldosterone

↓Addison's disease
↑Hyperaldosteronism — Primary
Secondary (edema states)

↓ Diuretics
↓ Tubulointerstitial diseases including ATN

Renal sodium reabsorption

↑ Renal failure
Edema states — Congestive heart failure
Cirrhotic liver disease
Nephrotic syndrome

Disordered regulation of body volume or osmolality causes changes in body sodium or water content, respectively. Depending on the ratio of these changes, hyponatremia or hypernatremia can occur, with or without a change in body volume. Generally, hyponatremia and hypernatremia reflect hypo-osmolality and hyperosmolality, respectively. To diagnose the cause of disordered sodium or water metabolism, try to establish body volume and osmolality.

Disordered water metabolism arises when *osmoregulation* is defective, resulting in too much or too little body water relative to the amount of body solute. As the main solute is sodium, too much water causes hyponatremia and too little causes hypernatremia. **Disordered sodium metabolism** arises when *volume regulation* is defective and there is inappropriate sodium retention or loss, causing the body volume to be too high or too low. **Mixed disorders** with abnormal volume and osmolality frequently occur and cause changes in both body sodium and water content.

Diagnosis is often difficult because initial pathologic changes are altered by compensatory mechanisms. Loss of isotonic salt solution from the gut, for example, causes hypovolemia and this triggers thirst. However, if the patient then ingests water without salt, hyponatremia will result. Indeed, most disorders of solute loss cause some secondary water retention as a result of ADH secretion and this can cause hypo-osmolality. Extrarenal loss of body sodium or water can occur from loss of body fluids such as blood, sweat, or gut secretions, especially diarrhea.

Disorders of water metabolism and osmolality control

Inadequate ADH action causes diabetes insipidus, whereas excess ADH action causes the syndrome of inappropriate ADH secretion (SIADH). Plasma hypo-osmolality normally suppresses ADH secretion and the minimum urine osmolality that can be produced is around 50 mosmol/kg H_2O. A urine concentration of 800 mosmol/kg H_2O is proof of normal ADH action.

Diabetes insipidus

Central diabetes insipidus occurs when the pituitary gland does not produce enough ADH. It can arise if the pituitary is damaged, particularly by trauma or a brain tumor.

Nephrogenic diabetes insipidus occurs when the kidney fails to respond to ADH. This can result from mutations in the V_2 ADH receptors or in the *AQP2* gene. It can also be a secondary effect of drugs, such as lithium, amphotericin or gentamicin, or it can arise in association with hypokalemia or hypercalcemia.

Clinically, there is polyuria and polydipsia. Plasma osmolality and sodium are high and urine osmolality and sodium low. Quite often, polydipsia and the high salt intake in Western diets maintain a normal plasma sodium and body volume despite the urinary losses. However, water deprivation fails to increase urine osmolality as it should.

In nephrogenic diabetes insipidus, ADH levels are high and there is no response to synthetic ADH. In central diabetes insipidus, ADH levels are low and synthetic ADH causes a rise in urine osmolality. Intranasal desmopressin (DDAVP), an ADH agonist, is therefore used as therapy for central diabetes insipidus.

Syndrome of inappropriate ADH secretion

Inappropriately high ADH levels cause excess water reabsorption by the kidney. This causes low plasma osmolality and low plasma sodium concentration. Urine is inappropriately concentrated for the low plasma osmolality. Causes include the stress-induced ADH secretion that can occur postoperatively and with lung cancers, especially the small cell type, which can secrete ADH. Treatment is by restriction of water intake because, even if there is excess ADH, the kidney continues to excrete some water and will eventually eliminate the excess water. Demeclocycline causes nephrogenic diabetes insipidus and is sometimes used to treat SIADH.

Psychogenic polydipsia

Massive abnormal water intake as a result of psychiatric disturbance can cause hypo-osmolality if water intake exceeds the capacity for its excretion.

Disorders of the volume regulatory mechanism and sodium metabolism

Inappropriate body volume control can occur if there is a primary abnormality of renal sodium handling. It can also occur when the kidney is normal, if there is an abnormality affecting the volume-sensing system, which drives inappropriate renal sodium handling.

Disorders causing excess sodium excretion

Addison's disease is caused by destruction of the adrenal glands, usually by an autoimmune process or tuberculosis. As sodium reabsorption in the distal tubule is promoted by aldosterone, a deficiency of this hormone causes hyponatremia. Hyperkalemia also occurs because potassium secretion is mechanistically linked to sodium reabsorption in the distal tubule. The excess sodium excretion causes hypovolemia. Glucocorticoid deficiency, if present, may also cause hypoglycemia. There may be generalized pigmentation probably caused by the melanocyte-stimulating side effects of excess ACTH produced by the pituitary, in an attempt to drive the adrenal gland. Autoimmune vitiligo can also occur. Treatment is with mineralocorticoid and glucocorticoid replacement.

Diuretics cause excess renal sodium excretion.

Intrinsic renal disease can cause renal salt wasting. Causes include tubulointerstitial disease because of its effects on tubular function and specific hereditary tubular conditions that affect renal salt handling (see Chapter 16).

Disorders causing inadequate sodium excretion

Excess aldosterone, whatever its cause, promotes excessive sodium reabsorption and enhanced potassium secretion in the distal tubule, causing hypernatremia and hypokalemia. Thirst is triggered, often causing polydipsia. Primary hyperaldosteronism is usually caused by an adrenal tumor or hyperplasia. Typically, plasma aldosterone levels are high and plasma renin levels low.

Renal failure ultimately reduces the ability of the kidney to excrete sodium or indeed other electrolytes. **The edema syndromes** (congestive heart failure, cirrhotic liver disease, and nephrotic syndrome) display a perceived reduction in body volume promotes both sodium and water conservation (see Chapter 20).

Hyponatremia and hypernatremia

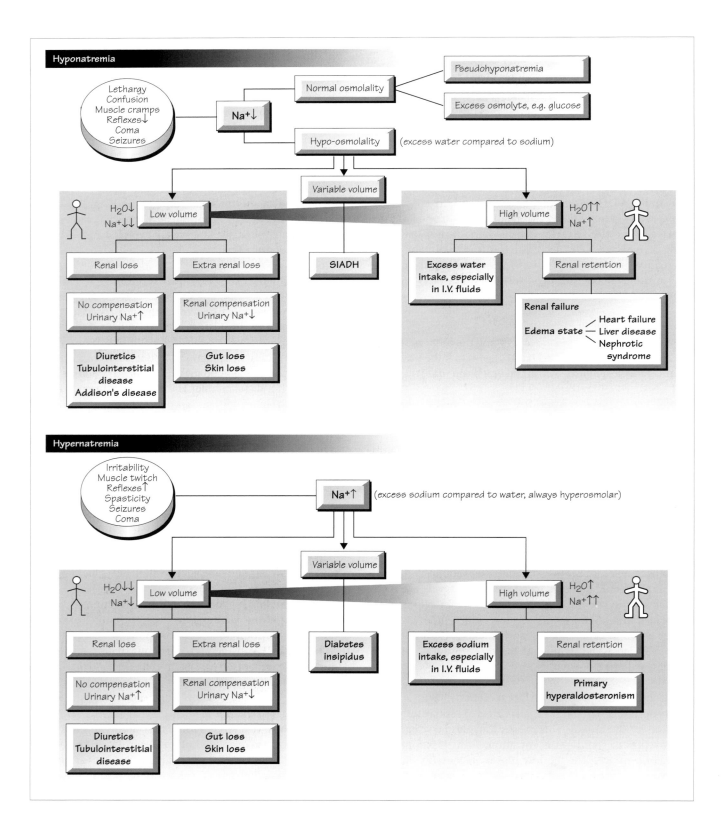

Abnormal plasma sodium concentration indicates an imbalance between the amount of sodium and water in the body. Hyponatremia is usually associated with hypo-osmolality and hypernatremia with hyperosmolality. Plasma and extravascular extracellular fluids are in equilibrium, so their sodium concentrations are the same. Sodium is the major extracellular osmolyte and changes in sodium concentration cause osmotic movement of water into or out of cells. This can impair cellular function, especially in the nervous system. Acute changes cause more severe symptoms than chronic changes. With chronic changes, the cells reduce the osmotic effect on them by altering intracellular osmolality. They do this by altering intracellular concentrations of ions and of urea and amino acids.

To assess hyponatremia or hypernatremia, evaluate body volume and consider all routes of fluid or electrolyte loss and gain. It can be helpful to establish whether the kidneys are acting appropriately to compensate for the sodium abnormality or acting inappropriately to exacerbate the changes. This is determined from whether the urine sodium concentration is appropriate for the body volume, plasma sodium concentration, and osmolality.

Hyponatremia

Hyponatremia always reflects hypo-osmolality unless there is pseudohyponatremia or an excess of another osmolyte in the plasma, such as glucose. Both these situations are easily diagnosed because measured plasma osmolality is normal. For example, an excess of glucose triggers a reduction in plasma sodium to maintain normal osmolality. Pseudohyponatremia occurs when there is an excess of protein or lipid in the plasma. Although the amount of sodium in each liter of plasma water is normal, the amount of water in each liter of total plasma is reduced because part of that volume of plasma is made up of the excess protein or lipid. Pseudohyponatremia is not a problem with modern ion-specific electrodes, which directly measure the sodium concentration in the aqueous phase.

True hyponatremia usually indicates excess water retention in relation to sodium. Apart from urine, body fluids are not usually hypertonic, so their loss does not cause hyponatremia directly. However, the loss of sodium and water in body fluids causes hypovolemia, which triggers non-osmotic ADH secretion. Hyponatremia can then follow if there is volume replacement with water which dilutes the body sodium and is retained as a result of the ADH.

Clinical features

Hyponatremia causes brain edema because water enters brain cells by osmosis. Mostly it is asymptomatic, but young and elderly people, menstruating women, and those with underlying neurologic conditions or other metabolic disorders are more vulnerable to symptoms. Clinical manifestations are initially those of depressed function, including lethargy, confusion, agitation, muscle cramps, nausea, and reduced tendon reflexes. Ultimately, seizures and coma can occur, particularly when sodium levels fall below 120 mmol/L. Mortality from hyponatremia can be high, but it is dangerous to correct hyponatremia too rapidly because this can cause neurological damage.

Treatment

Treatment of hyponatremia varies according to the body volume, but should include the correction of any underlying cause. If the body volume is high, treatment is restriction of fluid intake to reduce excess body water. Sometimes, diuretics can be useful, but they may exacerbate the hyponatremia. If body volume is low, the missing sodium and water should be replaced. During treatment, plasma sodium should be regularly checked to ensure that correction is not too rapid.

Hypernatremia

Hypernatremia usually results from a deficiency of body water relative to sodium, as happens in diabetes insipidus. Hypernatremia always causes hyperosmolality because sodium is the major extracellular ion. However, hyperosmolality can also result from excesses of other osmolytes, most commonly glucose in diabetes mellitus or urea in renal failure.

Most hypernatremia arises because of unreplaced water loss, so the body volume is usually low. The body's main defense against hypernatremia is therefore thirst. Thirst is often inadequate in elderly people or sick patients with no access to oral fluids. Hypernatremia can also result from excess aldosterone which causes excess sodium retention. Hypernatremia can occur if urine-concentrating mechanisms are inefficient and urine is dilute with a low sodium content. This occurs in diabetes insipidus and tubulointerstitial disease, and with diuretic use.

Clinical aspects

Hyperosmolality causes brain cells to shrink as water leaves them by osmosis. Various neurologic problems can occur including tearing of cerebral vessels. Early neurologic features are those of increased excitability including irritability, muscle twitches, brisk reflexes, and spasticity. Ultimately seizures and coma can occur. Children seem particularly vulnerable and mortality can be high.

Treatment

This includes correction of water deficits and prevention of ongoing loss, by correcting any underlying cause. Depending on the severity, replacement is with oral water or an intravenous 5% dextrose solution (the dextrose is removed by metabolism). As with hyponatremia, plasma sodium should be regularly checked during treatment to ensure that correction is not too rapid.

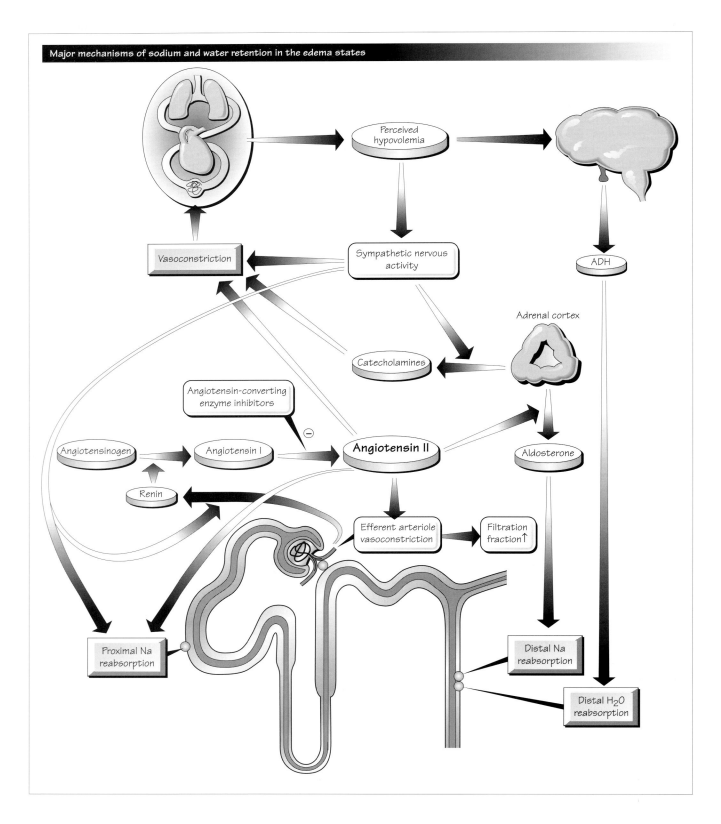

Normally, the high hydrostatic pressure of arterial blood entering tissue capillary beds causes some fluid to filter through the capillary wall into the interstitial space. Towards the venous end of the capillary bed hydrostatic pressure falls and the loss of fluid results in a rise in the plasma osmolality as a result of plasma proteins. These changes promote fluid movement back into the blood. Changes in capillary hydrostatic or osmotic pressure can cause **edema,** the accumulation of excess fluid in the interstitium. Venous obstruction or hypervolemia raises hydrostatic pressure at the venous end of the capillary bed, which reduces interstitial fluid reabsorption. A low plasma protein concentration lowers the capillary osmotic pressure and reduces interstitial fluid reabsorption.

Generalized edema occurs only when the body volume is too high. This can happen in advanced renal failure because the kidneys cannot excrete enough sodium or water. However, the major causes are congestive heart failure, cirrhotic liver disease, and nephrotic syndrome. In these conditions, renal sodium-handling mechanisms are intact, but the kidney receives neuroendocrine signals that promote sodium and water retention. This occurs because the volume sensors perceive that the circulation is under-filled and drive a volume-conserving response similar to that during hemorrhage. This response includes enhanced sympathetic and catecholamine activity, enhanced renin–angiotensin II–aldosterone activity, and excess antidiuretic hormone (ADH) secretion.

The afferent defect: perceived hypovolemia

Arterial baroreceptors are the dominant volume sensors, and monitor the stretching of arterial walls. In congestive heart failure, reduced cardiac output lowers the blood pressure which stimulates arterial baroreceptors. In cirrhotic liver disease, a fall in systemic vascular resistance lowers the blood pressure and triggers arterial baroreceptors. Low vascular resistance is caused by splanchnic vasodilation and the development of multiple arteriovenous shunts, including spider nevi in the skin. The vasodilation may be caused by either raised nitric oxide levels or a failure of the diseased liver to degrade other vasoactive substances. The volume-conserving response in nephrotic syndrome is less clearly understood. One possibility is that heavy proteinuria lowers plasma protein levels, allowing fluid to leak into the interstitium. The reduced circulating volume would then trigger a volume-conserving response.

The efferent volume-conserving response

Increased *sympathetic activity* mediated by α-adrenergic receptors promotes sodium reabsorption in the proximal tubule and reduces renal blood flow by renal vasoconstriction. This vasoconstriction, and any fall in the blood pressure, lower afferent arteriolar pressure, in turn promoting renin secretion. Stimulation of β-adrenergic receptors

also promotes renin release. A raised *angiotensin II* level causes further vasoconstriction and promotes proximal tubule sodium reabsorption. It also triggers *aldosterone* release, which increases distal tubular sodium reabsorption. The non-osmotic stimulation of *ADH* secretion promotes water retention and, if this is excessive in relation to the sodium retention, hyponatremia can occur. *Renal hemodynamics* may be relevant. A rise in the filtration fraction increases peritubular capillary osmotic pressure which promotes water and sodium reabsorption.

Hepatorenal syndrome. In severe liver disease, the efferent response can occasionally produce such a powerful vasoconstrictive effect that the GFR falls rapidly and acute renal failure occurs.

Location of edema

Edema fluid collects in slack tissues that are low in the body. Here, gravity causes a high hydrostatic venous pressure, opposing interstitial fluid reabsorption. Clinically, edema may be detectable in the lungs as pulmonary edema or as peripheral edema around the ankles, sacrum, and scrotum. Excess fluid can also accumulate as effusions, such as pleural effusions or ascites. In liver cirrhosis, hepatic fibrosis causes post-sinusoidal obstruction in the liver. This encourages fluid movement out of the liver and into the peritoneum as ascites.

Clinical aspects

High body volume usually raises the venous pressure, causing a high jugular venous pulse pressure. Outside the circulation, there is subcutaneous pitting edema—fluid moves away from a point where pressure is applied. Pulmonary edema can be heard with a stethoscope as fine inspiratory crackles.

Treatment

The primary disorder should be treated if possible. Edema may not need treatment unless it is impairing function. Initially, sodium restriction may be useful and water restriction is also appropriate if there is hyponatremia. Thiazide or loop **diuretics** promote sodium excretion and, if hypokalemia is a problem, potassium-sparing diuretics can be used. In heart failure, **angiotensin-converting enzyme inhibitors** are the first-line therapy because they block the vasoconstrictive and sodium-retaining actions of angiotensin II. The ascites of cirrhotic liver disease dissipates slowly, and large volumes are often drained percutaneously. Diuretics are given concurrently to reduce the reaccumulation of fluid, and intravenous albumin can be used to promote the retention of fluid in the circulation. As many cirrhotic patients have substantial hyperaldosteronism, potassium depletion is common and **spironolactone** reduces potassium loss.

21 Regulation of potassium metabolism

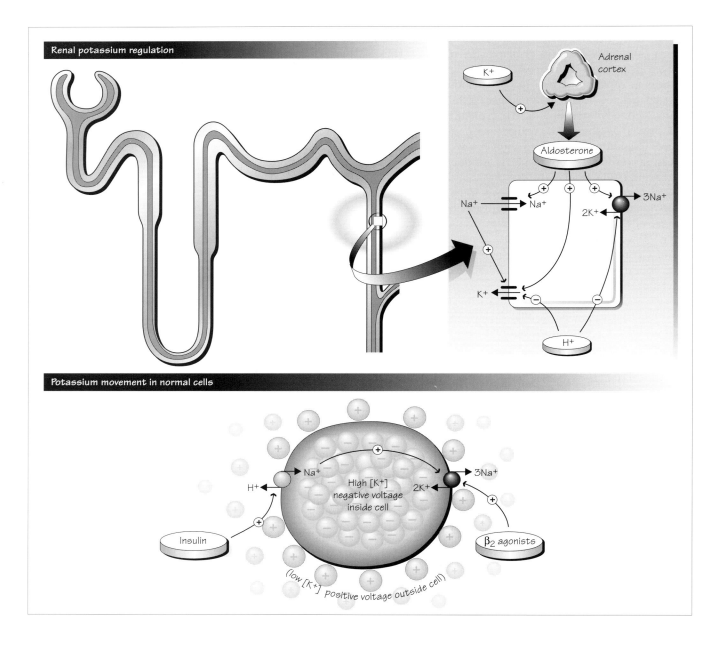

Renal potassium regulation

Adrenal cortex

K+

Aldosterone

Na+ → Na+

3Na+

2K+

K+

H+

Potassium movement in normal cells

Na+

H+

High [K+] negative voltage inside cell

3Na+

2K+

Insulin

β₂ agonists

(low [K+] positive voltage outside cell)

Potassium shifts across the cell membrane

The Na^+/K^+ ATPase pumps potassium into cells and the slow leak of K^+ out of cells through K^+ channels generates a negative potential inside all cells relative to the outside. This is the resting membrane potential from which the action potential starts in excitable cells. When extracellular potassium falls, the potassium gradient across the cell membrane is increased and this can activate sodium channels, triggering random action potentials. Hypokalemia can therefore cause enhanced neuronal excitability and cardiac dysrhythmias. Conversely, a rise in extracellular potassium reduces the potassium gradient, which inactivates sodium channels and tends to make membranes less excitable.

In both cases, the nature of any symptoms depends to some extent on the duration of the potassium abnormality and the rate of its development. Intracellular potassium levels do tend to change to compensate for the extracellular fluctuation. Chronic hypokalemia causes a shift of potassium out of the cells and chronic hyperkalemia a shift into them.

Influences on potassium movements across cell membranes

Insulin promotes Na^+/H^+ exchange across cell membranes and the rise in intracellular sodium promotes K^+ entry by the Na^+/K^+ ATPase.

β_2-Adrenergic agonists activate the Na^+/K^+ ATPase, so β blockade can increase plasma potassium whereas β agonists can reduce it.

pH. When H^+ ions enter the cells, they can displace K^+, so acidosis can raise plasma K^+ levels.

Thyroid hormones promote Na^+/K^+ ATPase synthesis and this can cause hypokalemia.

Renal potassium handling

The kidney and adrenal cortex regulate potassium levels, so abnormal potassium levels generally reflect renal or adrenal abnormalities. Homeostatic control of body potassium content is achieved by altering renal potassium handling. Although potassium reabsorption occurs mainly in the proximal tubule and thick ascending limb of the loop of Henle, the final potassium content of urine is controlled by potassium secretion in the cortical collecting duct.

The potassium channels in the cortical collecting duct are freely open for potassium movement, but movement of potassium into the filtrate requires a negative voltage in the lumen. This negative potential is generated by reabsorption of Na^+ through the ENaC channel, which is controlled by aldosterone. When sodium reabsorption is inhibited, as with amiloride, potassium secretion is less efficient. Conversely, enhanced delivery of sodium to the distal tubule promotes potassium secretion.

Control of renal potassium excretion

Renal potassium excretion increases in parallel with plasma potassium concentration. An increase in the potassium concentration of extracellular fluid increases the activity of the Na^+/K^+ ATPase at the basolateral surface of the principal cells of the cortical collecting ducts; this drives potassium secretion into the lumen. The reverse occurs when the plasma concentration falls. In addition, several other factors play important roles.

Aldosterone

A rise in the potassium concentration in the extracellular fluid of the adrenal cortex directly stimulates aldosterone release. In the cortical collecting duct, aldosterone promotes the synthesis of Na^+/K^+ ATPases and the insertion of more Na^+/K^+ ATPases into the basolateral membrane. Aldosterone also stimulates apical sodium and potassium channel activity, increasing sodium reabsorption and potassium secretion.

pH changes

Potassium secretion is reduced in acute acidosis and increased in acute alkalosis. A higher pH increases the apical potassium channel activity and the basolateral Na^+/K^+ ATPase activity—both changes that promote potassium secretion. With chronic changes in pH, compensatory changes can occur, but chronic metabolic acidosis is still usually associated with a low potassium level.

Flow rates

Increased flow rates in the collecting duct reduce potassium concentration in the lumen and, therefore, enhance potassium secretion (see Chapter 7).

Sodium delivery

If the sodium delivery to the collecting duct falls, there is less sodium reabsorption. This reduces sodium levels in principal cells, reducing the activity of the Na^+/K^+ ATPase, which lowers intracellular potassium levels and reduces the gradient for potassium secretion. Also, as described above, sodium reabsorption promotes the lumen-negative potential difference which drives potassium secretion.

Antidiuretic hormone (ADH)

This peptide reduces urinary flow rates but, to counteract the negative effect that this has on potassium secretion, ADH also stimulates apical potassium channel activity which helps to maintain potassium secretion at the correct level.

Drugs affecting potassium excretion

The most important drugs affecting potassium excretion are diuretics which increase urinary flow rates. The rise in the flow rate in the collecting ducts is the main factor in diuretic-induced potassium loss. Individual drugs have additional effects.

Thiazide diuretics reduce sodium and chloride reabsorption in the distal tubule. As potassium reabsorption in the distal tubule depends on sodium reabsorption, there is reduced potassium reabsorption.

Furosemide and the other loop diuretics inhibit the NaK2Cl co-transporter and so inhibit potassium reabsorption by this transporter.

Spironolactone antagonizes the effects of aldosterone and so reduces potassium secretion.

Amiloride, by blocking apical sodium entry into principal cells, reduces the concentration of intracellular sodium available for the Na^+/K^+ ATPase which normally drives potassium secretion.

Hypokalemia and hyperkalemia

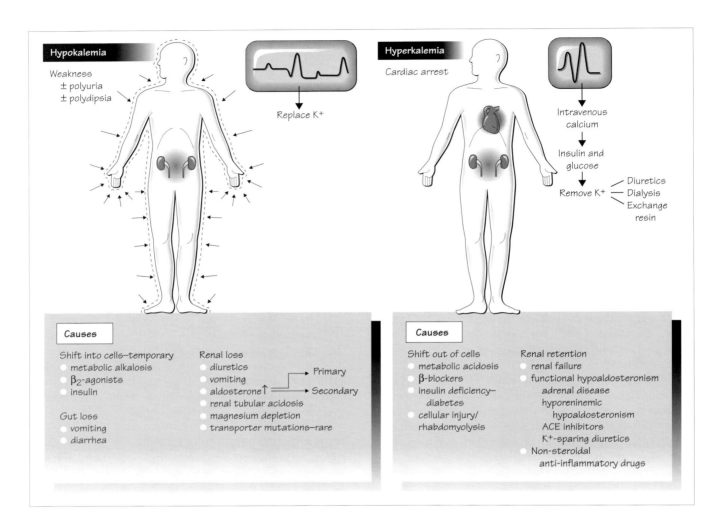

The normal plasma potassium concentration is 3.5–5.0 mmol/L. Abnormal plasma potassium levels can be life threatening. Potassium is the main determinant of the resting membrane potential of excitable cells and disturbances of plasma potassium can cause cardiac dysrhythmias or arrest. The distinction between the electrocardiographic (ECG) abnormalities produced by hypokalemia and hyperkalemia is critical and may be life-saving.

Hypokalemia

Hypokalemia usually reflects loss of potassium from the gut or kidney or, less commonly, a shift into the cells. In the kidneys, potassium loss can result from excess aldosterone or excess sodium delivery to the distal tubule, as can occur with loop or thiazide diuretic use. Excess aldosterone promotes potassium secretion and sodium reabsorption.

Causes

Loop diuretics, thiazide diuretics, and osmotic diuretics cause renal potassium excretion.

Hypokalemia associated with vomiting usually results from loss of potassium through the kidneys, rather than from the gut. Loss of acid gastric contents causes a metabolic alkalosis, which raises the plasma bicarbonate concentration and also the bicarbonate concentration in the filtrate. The excess sodium delivery to the distal tubule (as $NaHCO_3$) increases potassium secretion. There is often also volume depletion and aldosterone release, both of which further enhance potassium secretion.

Renal tubular acidoses can also cause hypokalemia. In proximal renal tubular acidosis, excess sodium delivery to the distal tubule as sodium bicarbonate increases potassium secretion. In distal renal tubular acidosis, more potassium is excreted to maintain electroneutrality because sodium is reabsorbed in the distal tubule.

Other causes of hypokalemia include the following.
• Acute stress such as that of acute myocardial infarction. This causes a β_2-adrenergic-receptor-mediated shift of potassium into cells.
• Insulin excess or overdose.
• Magnesium depletion. This reduces cellular potassium levels, probably by an effect on the Na^+/K^+ ATPase; it also causes renal potassium wasting. Potassium deficiency is difficult to correct if magnesium is deficient.
• Drugs such as penicillins, aminoglycosides, and amphotericin can cause renal potassium loss.
• Mutations in the distal tubule NaCl co-transporter, the NaK2Cl co-transporter in the loop of Henle or the ENaC channel in the collecting duct (see Chapter 16).
• Hypokalemic periodic paralysis is a rare autosomal dominant disorder characterized by periodic attacks of paralysis associated with hypokalemia.

Clinical features
Symptoms are unusual unless the potassium level is very low. There may be muscle weakness, constipation, or gut ileus. Polyuria and compensatory polydipsia can occur as a result of renal antidiuretic hormone (ADH) resistance. Hypokalemia predisposes to digitalis toxicity.

ECG changes
Hypokalemia increases automaticity and delays repolarization of cardiac cells. This predisposes the heart to dysrhythmias such as ectopic beats, atrioventricular block, and atrial and ventricular fibrillation. The classic changes are progressive lengthening of the P–R interval, S-T segment depression, flattening of the T waves, and an increase in the U wave.

Treatment
Potassium administration, usually as oral or intravenous potassium chloride, is the usual treatment. If a metabolic alkalosis is present, potassium bicarbonate can be given. If the problem is caused by a diuretic, a potassium-sparing diuretic can be added.

Hyperkalemia
Hyperkalemia usually represents reduced urinary potassium secretion or less commonly acute release from cells or a failure to enter cells. Hyperkalemia does not persist unless there is impaired renal excretion. Remember that, if cells in a blood sample are hemolysed, intracellular potassium has been released into the plasma and this can cause a spuriously elevated plasma potassium estimation.

Causes
Shifts out of cells. During metabolic acidosis, H^+ ions enter cells to be buffered and K^+ ions leave the cells to maintain electroneutrality. Insulin deficiency in diabetic ketoacidosis allows the net movement of potassium out of the cells. Rhabdomyolysis or tissue destruction, or lysis such as that caused by chemotherapy, can cause massive potassium loss from cells.

Failure of renal secretion. In renal failure, potassium accumulates because of the reduced number of nephrons capable of potassium excretion.

Other causes of hyperkalemia include the following.
• Trimethoprim and pentamidine therapy. Both can block potassium secretion in the collecting tubule.
• Hypoaldosteronism. The hyperkalemia can result from inadequate renin release, inadequate aldosterone release, or tubular resistance to aldosterone. Hypoaldosteronism is usually caused by potassium-sparing diuretics or hyporeninemic hypoaldosteronism. The latter usually arises in diabetic nephropathy when there is a reduced glomerular filtration rate and reduced renin secretion.

Clinical features
Symptoms, if present, include muscle weakness and cardiac dysrhythmias. The key cardiac dysrhythmia—ventricular fibrillation—causes cardiac arrest.

ECG changes
The typical ECG changes of hyperkalemia are loss of P waves, widening of the QRS complex, loss of the S-T segment, and tall wide T waves. As the potassium level rises, the changes take on a sine wave appearance. The first change is the appearance of a narrowed, peaked T wave (this represents rapid repolarization); then the QRS widens into the T wave and the P wave is lost.

Treatment
The patient should be placed on a cardiac monitor. If there are ECG changes, urgent treatment is essential.
• Initially, calcium, given as calcium gluconate or calcium chloride, will antagonize the effects of potassium on the cardiac action potential, but this is short-lived.
• In the intermediate term, potassium can be shifted into cells by administering insulin, combined with glucose, to prevent hypoglycemia. β_2 Agonists can also be used for this purpose. Administration of sodium bicarbonate produces a temporary alkalosis which also promotes the intracellular movement of potassium.
• In the longer term, excess potassium must be removed from the body. Diuretics, such as furosemide, combined with hydration encourage renal excretion. If renal function is severely impaired, dialysis or hemofiltration will remove potassium. Cation exchange resins such as sodium polystyrene sulfonate can be given orally or rectally and bind potassium in the gut, exchanging it for sodium.

Regulation of divalent ions and disorders of phosphate and magnesium

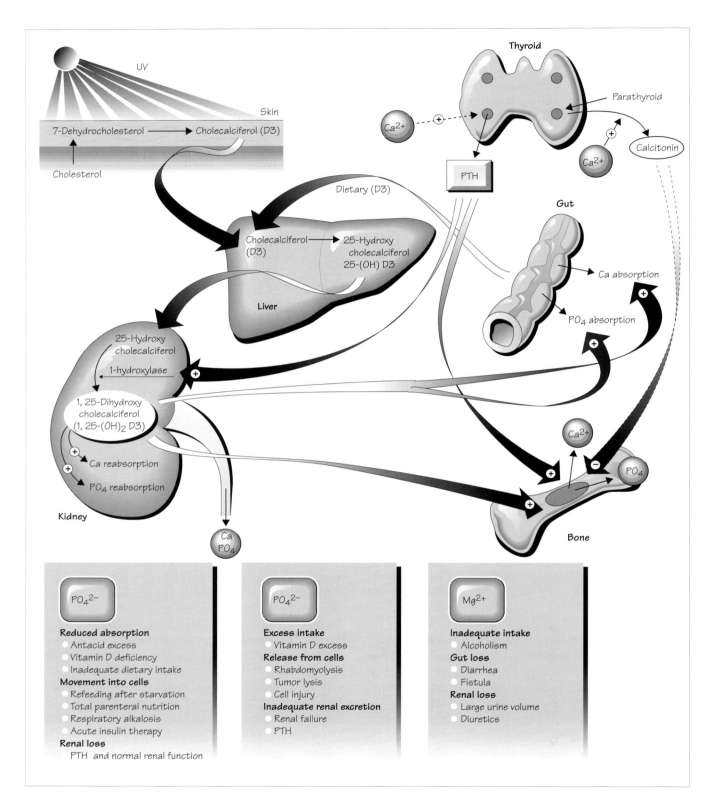

Control of calcium and phosphate

Parathyroid hormone

Parathyroid hormone (PTH) is a protein secreted by the chief cells of the parathyroid gland, when extracellular ionized calcium levels fall. A calcium-sensing protein on the surface of chief cells influences PTH release. PTH receptors in the bone and kidneys act via G proteins to activate adenyl cyclase and raise cAMP levels. Excess PTH increases serum calcium and reduces serum phosphate.

- **In bone**, PTH stimulates bone-building osteoblasts which themselves stimulate bone-resorbing osteoclasts. There is net bone resorption with calcium and phosphate release.
- **In the kidney**, PTH has three effects: (i) it increases vitamin D synthesis; (ii) it reduces proximal tubular phosphate reabsorption which increases phosphate excretion; and (iii) it increases distal tubular calcium reabsorption by activating calcium channels.

Vitamin D

Dietary cholecalciferol is absorbed in the small intestine or synthesized in the skin by the action of ultraviolet light. The liver converts cholecalciferol to 25-hydroxycholecalciferol. This is converted by 1α-hydroxylase in the cells of the renal proximal tubule to 1,25-dihydroxycholecalciferol, the principal active form of vitamin D. Vitamin D acts on receptors in the gut, bone, and kidney to raise levels of both calcium and phosphate. The major effect is in the gut, where calcium and phosphate absorption are increased. Vitamin D enhances the action of PTH, promoting net bone resorption with calcium and phosphate release. Vitamin D stimulates renal calcium and phosphate reabsorption. The vitamin D receptor acts as a transcription factor, increasing levels of calbindins in the distal tubule cells.

Calcitonin and other hormones

Calcitonin is a peptide secreted by the C cells of the thyroid gland when ionized calcium levels in the plasma fall. It reduces osteoclast activity, but its role is unclear. Growth hormone (acting via insulin-like growth factor 1 or IGF-1), insulin, and thyroxine promote renal phosphate reabsorption, whereas corticosteroids and chronic acidosis inhibit phosphate reabsorption.

Hypophosphatemia

Severe hypophosphatemia indicates phosphate deficiency, but moderate hypophosphatemia is often the result of movement of phosphate into cells. Movement into cells occurs if intracellular phosphate is used up to generate phosphorylated metabolic products, such as glucose 6-phosphate and ATP. Plasma phosphate can fall if glycolysis increases suddenly, as with re-feeding after starvation, starting total parenteral nutrition, giving insulin in diabetic ketoacidosis, or with respiratory alkalosis. Hypophosphatemia occurs with alcohol-related malnutrition and with ingestion of phosphate-binding antacids. PTH promotes phosphaturia, so hyperparathyroidism of any type can cause hypophosphatemia if renal function is not impaired. Vitamin D deficiency impairs calcium and phosphate absorption in the gut, lowering both plasma levels of both calcium and phosphate. Severe phosphate deficiency lowers cellular ATP levels which can impair cellular function.

Clinical features include weakness of skeletal, cardiac, and smooth muscle, causing dysphagia, ileus, inadequate respiratory muscle strength, and impaired myocardial contractility. Neurologic problems include paresthesia, confusion, seizures, and coma. *Treatment* is with oral sodium phosphate or potassium phosphate. Intravenous phosphate can cause severe hypocalcemia and is used only with severe phosphate depletion.

Hyperphosphatemia

Hyperphosphatemia can result from reduced urinary phosphate excretion, excessive phosphate intake, or phosphate release from cells. Renal failure is the commonest cause of severe hyperphosphatemia. As PTH promotes phosphate excretion, hypoparathyroidism can cause hyperphosphatemia. Excess vitamin D promotes excess phosphate absorption in the gut and hyperphosphatemia. Chemotherapy, tumor lysis, and rhabdomyolysis all release phosphate from cells.

Clinical features include those of hypocalcemia if it is present, such as tetany. If phosphate is elevated and calcium is not low, soft tissue calcification can occur. *Treatment* is by hydration with saline which promotes phosphaturia if renal function is normal (see also Chapter 41).

Hypomagnesemia and hypermagnesemia

Magnesium is required by many essential enzymes and stabilizes excitable cell membranes, including those in the heart. Intracellular magnesium can regulate both K^+ and Ca^{2+} channels, and promotes intracellular potassium retention by stimulating the Na^+/K^+ ATPase.

Hypomagnesemia is usually caused by magnesium loss from the gut or kidneys or inadequate intake especially in people with alcohol problems. Clinically, symptoms are neurologic and muscular, resembling those of hypocalcemia. There may be tetany, Chvostek's sign, and Trousseau's sign (see Chapter 24), seizures, and cardiac dysrhythmias, especially ventricular dysrhythmias. ECG changes include a prolonged P–R interval, QRS widening, T-wave inversion, and prominent U waves. Treatment is with oral or intravenous magnesium chloride.

Hypermagnesemia is rare and is usually the result of excess magnesium intake or administration. Clinical features include bradycardia, hypotension, reduced consciousness, and respiratory depression. Treatment involves removal of excess magnesium, using furosemide and hydration or dialysis. Calcium administration reverses some of the dangerous effects of magnesium on the heart.

24 Hypocalcemia and hypercalcemia

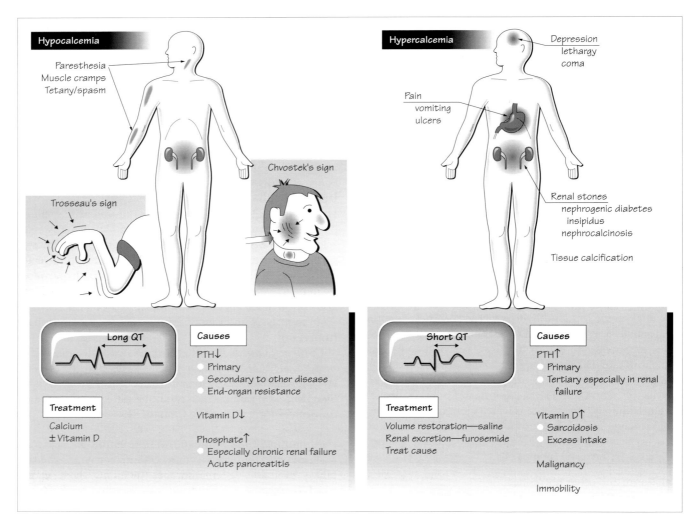

Around 40% of serum calcium is protein bound, but it is the concentration of free calcium ions that is biologically relevant. Changes in protein concentration alter the total calcium concentration, but the free calcium ion concentration usually remains normal. An increase in H^+ or a very large increase in Na^+ can displace Ca^{2+} ions from their binding sites on proteins. There are algorithms to estimate these effects but, if there is doubt, the free Ca^{2+} should be measured directly.

Hypocalcemia
Causes
Vitamin D deficiency
Vitamin D deficiency can result from inadequate nutrition, inadequate sun exposure, or renal damage. It causes hypocalcemia and hypophosphatemia. Vitamin D is fat soluble, and fat malabsorption as a result of pancreatic, biliary, or small intestinal disease can cause vitamin D deficiency. Vitamin D-dependent rickets is an autosomal recessive disorder caused by a deficiency of renal 1α-hydroxylase.

Hypoparathyroidism
Primary hypoparathyroidism can be sporadic and idiopathic. Familial forms result from mutations in the parathyroid hormone (PTH) gene or the DiGeorge syndrome of underdeveloped parathyroid and thymic tissues. **Secondary hypoparathyroidism** describes parathyroid damage that is secondary to another disease process. Causes include iron deposition in thalassemia, copper deposition in Wilson's disease, or autoimmune diseases involving several endocrine organs (especially the adrenals). **Pseudohypoparathyroidism** is a rare genetic defect. Cells do not respond to PTH because of deficiency in the G protein, which stimulates adenyl cyclase. Clinical features include

hypocalcemia, hyperphosphatemia, learning disorders, short stature, and abnormally short metacarpal and metatarsal bones. Pseudo-pseudohypoparathyroidism is a condition with the same phenotype but no biochemical abnormalities.

Hyperphosphatemia and other causes
Hyperphosphatemia causes hypocalcemia by forming calcium phosphate complexes which are deposited in bone or other tissues. Acute pancreatitis lowers serum calcium, probably because calcium forms soap-like precipitates with lipid derivatives in the peritoneum. Rarely, bone-forming malignancies such as prostatic and breast cancer can sequester calcium in bone.

Clinical features
There is neuromuscular irritability with paresthesia, circumoral numbness, muscle cramps, tetany, laryngospasm, and sometimes seizures or psychosis. Chvostek's and Trousseau's signs may be present. *Chvostek's* sign is a facial muscle twitch when the facial nerve is tapped below the zygomatic bone. *Trousseau's* sign is a spasm with hyperextended fingers and metacarpophalangeal flexion, when a sphygmomanometer cuff is inflated for 3 min around the upper arm. Cardiac abnormalities include a *prolonged Q–T interval*, peaked T waves, and rarely ventricular fibrillation or heart block.

Treatment
Treat symptomatic acute hypocalcemia with intravenous calcium gluconate or calcium chloride. Chronic hypocalcemia can be treated with oral calcium replacement, which can be supplemented with vitamin D. Magnesium levels must be corrected if low. Thiazides can raise calcium levels.

If phosphate levels are high, phosphate should be lowered, to avoid calcium phosphate deposition in tissues when calcium is given.

Hypercalcemia
Causes
Hyperparathyroidism
Primary hyperparathyroidism is the most common cause of hypercalcemia, especially in elderly women. The usual cause is primary hyperplasia or a single parathyroid adenoma. Adenomas can be familial. Adenomas are associated with other endocrine abnormalities, including the multiple endocrine neoplasia (MEN) syndromes. Treatment involves surgical removal of parathyroid tissue. In **secondary hyperparathyroidism,** the calcium level is low and excess PTH is an appropriate response to correct the low calcium. **Tertiary hyperparathyroidism** is the situation following long-standing secondary hyperparathyroidism, in which the parathyroid glands continue to secrete excess PTH autonomously, even when calcium levels have risen.

Continued PTH secretion causes a high calcium level as in primary hyperparathyroidism.

Malignancy
This is the second most common cause of hypercalcemia. Typical causes are squamous cell lung carcinoma, metastatic breast carcinoma, or kidney, ovary, and hematologic malignancies (especially myeloma). Hypercalcemia arises because of local bone erosion and because tumors can produce a PTH analogue, PTH-related peptide (PTHrP) and osteoclast-activating cytokines.

Excess vitamin D and other causes
In lymphomas and granulomatous diseases such as sarcoidosis, tuberculosis, and leprosy, macrophages can synthesize vitamin D which can lead to hypercalcemia. Excess thyroid hormones can increase osteoclast bone resorption, causing hypercalcemia. Adrenocortical insufficiency can cause hypercalcemia. Immobilization causes bone resorption. Rapid bone turnover in Paget's disease can cause hypercalcemia. Excess calcium ingestion as milk and alkali, to relieve peptic ulcer symptom, causes milk–alkali syndrome with deposition of calcium phosphate. Thiazide diuretics reduce urinary calcium excretion. Mutations in the calcium-sensing receptor on parathyroid cells cause familial hypocalciuric hypercalcemia.

Clinical features
Mild hypercalcemia is usually asymptomatic. Higher levels cause neurologic, gastrointestinal, and renal symptoms ('depressive moans, abdominal groans, renal stones'). There may be drowsiness, lethargy, weakness, depression, and coma. There is often constipation, nausea, vomiting, anorexia, and peptic ulceration. Calcium causes nephrogenic diabetes insipidus, producing dehydration. Sustained hypercalcemia can cause renal stone formation and nephrocalcinosis. Severe chronic hypercalcemia can cause tissue calcification, which may be detectable radiographically or as visible corneal calcification.

ECG changes include *shortening of the Q–T interval*, sometimes with broad T waves and atrioventricular block. Hypercalcemia can potentiate digitalis toxicity.

Treatment
Sodium and water losses should be replaced with intravenous saline to restore body volume and to encourage renal calcium excretion. Loop diuretics can be used to increase the urinary excretion of calcium. Thiazide diuretics should be stopped. Bisphosphonates stabilize bone and inhibit osteoclast action, thus preventing bone resorption. They are useful in malignancy-associated hypercalcemia. Steroids block osteoclast-activating cytokines and are helpful in malignancy and sarcoidosis. If there is excess PTH, surgery to remove parathyroid tissue is appropriate.

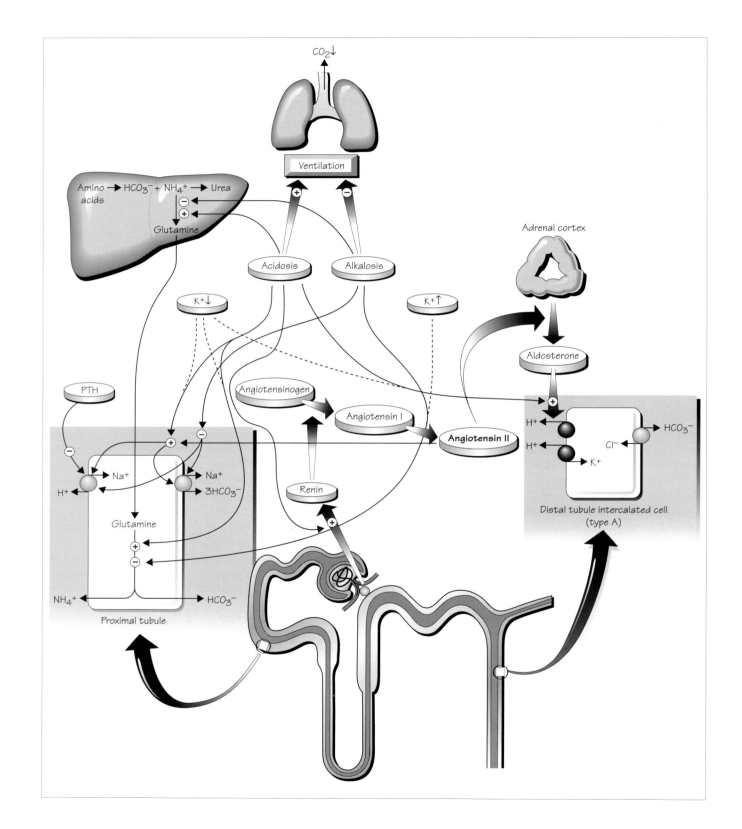

Total body pH can be regulated by controlling the ratio of CO_2 (acid) to HCO_3^- (base) in plasma.

Ventilation controls the CO_2 level and the kidney controls the HCO_3^- level. Disorders of acid–base metabolism can therefore arise either from excess acid or base, or from diseases altering CO_2 or HCO_3^- levels. In a respiratory acid–base disturbance, the primary disorder alters the CO_2 level whereas, in a metabolic acid–base disturbance, the primary disorder alters the HCO_3^- level either directly or by the addition of acid or base to the body. In a mixed disorder, there may be both respiratory and metabolic disturbances. When HCO_3^- or CO_2 levels change, the pH can be brought back toward normal by altering the other buffer partner in the same direction (see Chapter 8).

Renal responses to acid–base abnormalities

Metabolic acidosis

With metabolic acidosis, plasma and filtrate bicarbonate concentrations are low. Acidosis directly stimulates proximal tubular glutamine metabolism, which produces NH_4^+ for urinary excretion and generates new bicarbonate. In addition, acidosis increases H^+ secretion and therefore bicarbonate reabsorption in both the proximal and distal tubule. In the proximal tubule, there is increased synthesis of the apical Na^+/H^+ exchangers and increased activity of the basolateral $Na^+/3HCO_3^-$ co-transporters. In the distal tubule, there are increased numbers of H^+ ATPases in the apical membranes of type A intercalated cells. Acidosis directly stimulates renin release, which raises angiotensin II production, and aldosterone secretion, which also promotes H^+ ATPase activity in type A intercalated cells.

Metabolic alkalosis

Bicarbonate levels are high in metabolic alkalosis and this inhibits renal ammoniagenesis. The renal response to alkalosis depends on **chloride**. Low chloride levels exacerbate metabolic alkalosis. In the collecting duct, active secretion of H^+ by the H^+ ATPase is associated with passive co-transport of chloride to maintain electroneutrality. If plasma and therefore filtrate chloride levels are low, the gradient for chloride movement into the filtrate is increased. This enhances H^+ ion secretion and with it bicarbonate reabsorption. In the collecting tubule, type B intercalated cells secrete bicarbonate in exchange for chloride ions and bicarbonate secretion is inhibited if chloride levels are low.

Respiratory acidosis and alkalosis

In **acute respiratory acidosis**, excess CO_2 shifts the carbonic anhydrase reaction toward HCO_3^- production and there is a slight increase in HCO_3^-. However, in chronic respiratory acidosis, there is enhanced bicarbonate reabsorption in the proximal and distal tubules. In the proximal tubule, there is increased apical Na^+/H^+ exchange and basolateral $Na^+/3HCO_3^-$ co-transport. In the distal tubule, there is H^+ ATPase insertion and enhanced expression of the HCO_3^-/Cl^- exchanger.

In **respiratory alkalosis**, the changes are the opposite of those in respiratory acidosis and plasma bicarbonate levels fall as a result of reduced renal bicarbonate reabsorption. Low CO_2 levels also trigger an acute mild increase in lactic and citric acid production.

Role of the liver in acid–base metabolism

The hepatic catabolism of proteins that contain sulfur and PO_4^{3-} generates acid. Most other hepatic protein catabolism is neutral and produces both HCO_3^- and NH_4^+. Most of the NH_4^+ reacts with the HCO_3^- or forms urea and has no impact on acid–base balance. However, some of the NH_4^+ is diverted to hepatic glutamine synthesis. The glutamine travels in the blood to the proximal tubule for renal ammoniagenesis. Each NH_4^+ excreted in the kidney is associated with one new HCO_3^- added to the blood. Both hepatic glutamine synthesis and renal ammoniagenesis are enhanced by acidosis and reduced by alkalosis.

Role of the lungs in acid–base metabolism

As CO_2 diffuses well and is highly soluble, there is a relatively linear relationship between ventilation and plasma CO_2 levels. A fall in pH triggers arterial chemoreceptors, particularly in the carotid body, and increases the ventilation rate.

Effects of potassium on acid–base disorders

Acidosis causes H^+ ions to enter cells and potassium ions exit to maintain electroneutrality. Thus, *acidosis can cause hyperkalemia and alkalosis can cause hypokalemia*. In addition:

• hyperkalemia promotes acidosis. Potassium inhibits proximal tubule NH_4^+ production and, in the loop of Henle, K^+ competes with NH_4^+ at the NaK2Cl co-transporter, impairing NH_4^+ excretion; and
• hypokalemia promotes alkalosis. Potassium depletion enhances proximal NH_4^+ production, Na^+/H^+ exchange, and the activity of the $Na^+/3HCO_3^-$ co-transporter. Low intracellular potassium levels stimulate the collecting duct H^+/K^+ ATPase, promoting H^+ secretion, K^+ reabsorption, and HCO_3^- reabsorption.

Hormonal effects

Aldosterone increases acid secretion by the H^+ ATPase in type A intercalated cells in the distal tubule. **Angiotensin II** upregulates the Na^+/H^+ exchangers and $Na^+/3HCO_3^-$ co-transporter and therefore promotes H^+ secretion and bicarbonate reabsorption. **Parathyroid hormone** (PTH) stimulates proximal ammoniagenesis, and decreases proximal bicarbonate reabsorption by inhibiting Na^+/H^+ exchange. **Renal nerves** and **catecholamines** also stimulate the Na^+/H^+ exchangers, promoting alkalosis.

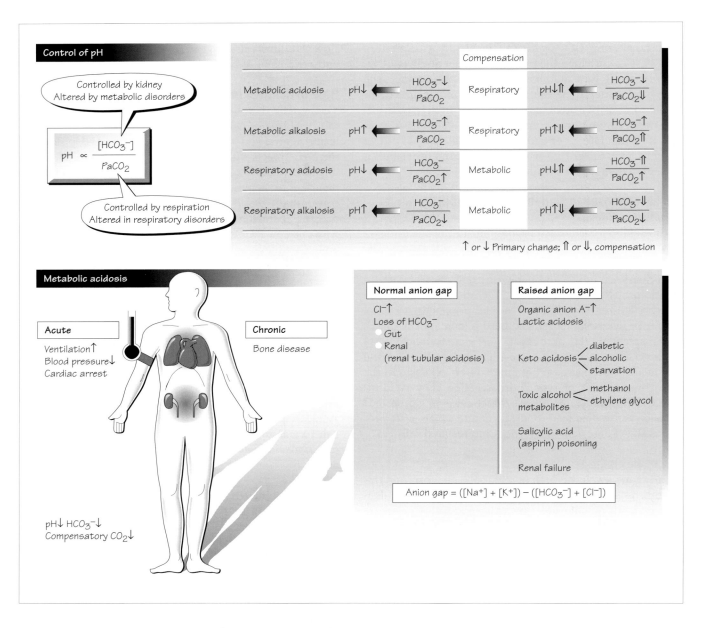

Acid–base disorders can seem confusing, but there are only a few common disorders and they are relatively easy to distinguish. It is essential to establish the nature of the disturbance before trying to determine the cause. To do this, the following questions are useful.

- Is the patient acidotic or alkalotic? This is determined by the **arterial pH**.
- Is ventilation compensating for the pH change or contributing to it? This is determined by the **arterial $P\text{co}_2$** and distinguishes metabolic from respiratory disorders, respectively.

- If there is a metabolic acidosis, is the **anion gap normal or elevated**? This determines whether acid has been acquired or bicarbonate lost.
- Last, what is the diagnosis?

Metabolic acidosis

Metabolic acidosis arises from the gain of acid or the loss of base as bicarbonate.

Clinical features

Acidotic patients have increased ventilation, which can be

deep and rapid (Kussmaul's respiration). At low pH, the blood pressure falls as a result of reduced peripheral resistance and impaired myocardial contractility, resulting from poor actin–myosin cross-bridge cycling. Pulmonary edema and, ultimately, ventricular arrest can occur. Chronic metabolic acidosis causes hypercalciuria and buffering of acid by bone causes loss of calcium from the bone. Serum potassium is often elevated, as a result of a shift of potassium out of the cells. In *pure metabolic acidosis,* the pH is low, HCO_3^- is low and P_{CO_2} is low to compensate.

The anion gap in metabolic acidosis

The **anion gap** is the difference between the measured cations and the measured anions in plasma. As plasma is always electrically neutral, this difference is made up by unmeasured anions. These are usually proteins, organic acids, sulfate, and phosphate, and the normal anion gap is around 6–16 mmol/L. In metabolic acidosis:

• an increased anion gap occurs if a new acid is added to the body. This dissociates producing free H^+ (which uses up bicarbonate) and anions (which take the place of the bicarbonate); and

• a normal anion gap occurs if there is simple loss of bicarbonate. This causes a compensatory rise in plasma chloride concentration, so the anion gap is normal.

$$\textbf{Anion gap} = \left(\left[Na^+\right]+\left[K^+\right]\right)-\left(\left[HCO_3^-\right]+\left[Cl^-\right]\right)$$

Causes of normal anion gap metabolic acidosis
Gut bicarbonate loss
Bicarbonate can be lost from the gut in diarrhea, or from the small intestinal, pancreatic, or biliary drains, and from fistulae. Ileal conduits that divert urine to the bowel, especially ureterosigmoidostomies, cause acidosis because the bowel mucosa exchanges chloride in the urine for bicarbonate.

Renal bicarbonate loss
Loss of bicarbonate in the urine causes acidosis and is the basis of some renal tubular acidoses (see Chapter 28).

Causes of increased anion gap metabolic acidosis
Addition of acid
Lactic acid is the end-product of anerobic metabolism and is normally metabolized to bicarbonate by the liver in an oxygen-dependent pathway. It accumulates when there is reduced oxygen delivery to the tissues, impaired oxidative metabolism, or reduced liver function. Lactic acidosis usually occurs in very sick, hemodynamically shocked, or septic patients and indicates inadequate tissue oxygenation, often combined with impaired lactate metabolism caused by poor liver perfusion.

The ketoacids, β-hydroxybutyric acid and acetoacetic acid, accumulate during diabetic ketoacidosis and are present in blood and urine. The absence of insulin promotes their production and inhibits their catabolism. In people with non-insulin-dependent (type 2) diabetes, the small amount of insulin present prevents these changes. Alcoholic ketoacidosis and starvation also produce excess plasma and urine ketones. Alcoholic ketoacidosis probably represents a combination of alcohol toxicity and starvation.

Toxic alcohols such as methanol and ethylene glycol (antifreeze) cause a difference between the predicted osmolality (calculated from the concentrations of ions, glucose, and urea) and the measured osmolality. In both cases, alcohol dehydrogenase metabolizes the alcohol to a more seriously toxic metabolite. This can be prevented by saturating the enzyme with ethanol, while the poisonous alcohol is removed by dialysis. Methanol typically causes abdominal pain, vomiting, headache, and visual disturbances or blindness resulting from severe retinitis. Ethylene glycol causes similar symptoms to methanol, as well as acute and chronic renal failure, but not usually retinitis.

Aspirin poisoning triggers increased ventilation, causing an early respiratory alkalosis. However, salicylic acid itself then causes a metabolic acidosis. There is often tinnitus and nausea, hyperventilation and sometimes non-cardiogenic pulmonary edema and an elevated prothrombin time. Seizures and death can occur if cerebral tissue levels are high.

Rare inborn errors of metabolism, such as the aminoacidemias, can produce metabolic acidosis presenting after birth.

Failure of acid excretion
Acute or chronic renal failure leads to the retention of phosphate, sulfate, and organic anions. Initially there is buffering by bicarbonate and then also by bone and intracellular buffers.

Treatment of metabolic acidosis
The primary abnormality should be corrected. Acute intravenous bicarbonate administration can worsen intracellular acidosis by producing CO_2 which diffuses into cells and lowers the intracellular pH. Excess acid should be removed, either by further metabolism in the case of lactate and ketones, or by urinary excretion or dialysis for other acids. Slow bicarbonate administration will correct the bicarbonate deficiency in hyperchloremic metabolic acidosis.

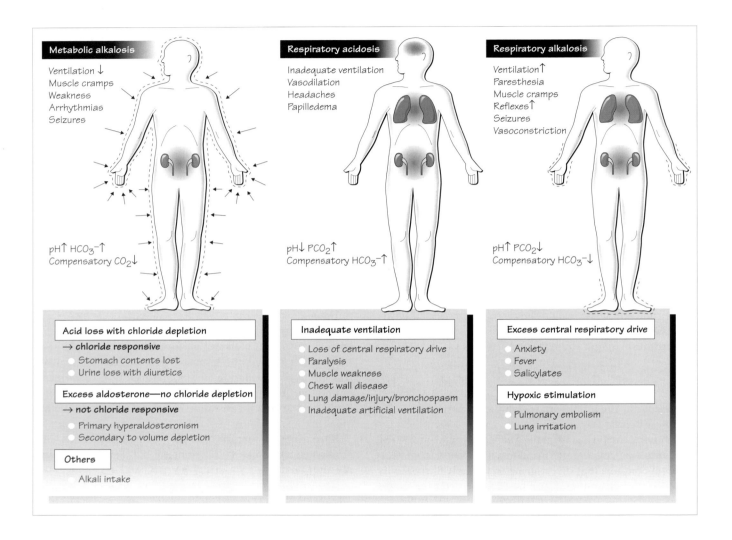

Metabolic alkalosis

In metabolic alkalosis, plasma pH and plasma bicarbonate levels are both raised. This can result from addition of bicarbonate to the blood or from loss of H^+ ions from the body. As plasma bicarbonate rises above a certain level, the concentration of bicarbonate in the filtrate exceeds the tubular threshold for bicarbonate reabsorption and the excess bicarbonate is excreted. For this reason, a severe metabolic alkalosis can arise only when the kidneys cannot excrete this excess bicarbonate. This can happen if there is inadequate renal perfusion or excess aldosterone. **Aldosterone** enhances distal bicarbonate reabsorption in type A-intercalated cells by stimulating the H^+ ATPase. Aldosterone also promotes sodium reabsorption in the distal tubule which increases potassium loss. The hypokalemia further enhances bicarbonate reabsorption (see Chapter 25).

Factors that worsen metabolic alkalosis

Low plasma chloride

Chloride is necessary for bicarbonate excretion and if plasma chloride concentration is low, chloride replacement is necessary to achieve efficient bicarbonate excretion. Aldosterone excess is not associated with a low chloride concentration and chloride replacement is of no benefit.

Hypovolemia

This exacerbates metabolic alkalosis by stimulating aldosterone release which increases bicarbonate reabsorption as discussed above.

Causes of metabolic alkalosis

Loss of acid from the gut or kidney

Gastric contents are acidic because the luminal,

omeprazole-inhibited H^+ ATPase in parietal cells secretes acid into the stomach. Loss of gastric contents, particularly when there is repeated vomiting, as in pyloric stenosis, can cause metabolic alkalosis. There is often also volume depletion and chloride loss.

Addition of bicarbonate to the body
This can result from the ingestion or administration of bicarbonate or substances such as lactate, citrate, or acetate, which are metabolized to generate bicarbonate.

Renal dysfunction and aldosterone
Any cause of a high aldosterone level can cause a metabolic alkalosis by increasing H^+ ATPase activity and therefore bicarbonate reabsorption in the distal tubule.

Other causes
Diuretics can contribute to alkalosis by causing hypovolemia with secondary hyperaldosteronism, hypokalemia, and chloride depletion. Glycyrrhizinic acid in black licorice causes a hypokalemic metabolic alkalosis and hypertension by upregulating renal mineralocorticoid receptors, thereby enhancing the effect of aldosterone. Severe potassium depletion can cause metabolic alkalosis by its effect on the kidney. Rare causes of metabolic alkalosis include excess citrate administration in blood products, and milk–alkali syndrome (see Chapter 24).

Clinical features
These are not specific but can include muscle cramps, weakness, dysrhythmias, and seizures. These features may relate to a reduction in free calcium that can occur when calcium ions bind to the negative charges on proteins at sites normally occupied by H^+. The normal respiratory response to metabolic alkalosis is diminished breathing, but obviously the hypoxic drive to breathing ensures that breathing maintains oxygenation adequately. There is usually hypokalemia as a result of the shift of potassium into cells.

If the underlying cause is not clinically obvious, vomiting, diuretic overuse, and primary hyperaldosteronism should be considered. Vomiting and diuretics lead to volume contraction whereas excess mineralocorticoid leads to volume expansion.

Treatment
The underlying cause should be treated. Chloride-responsive alkalosis responds to chloride and volume replacement and improved renal hemodynamics. The increase in chloride delivery promotes distal bicarbonate secretion. Hypokalemia should be corrected. In non-chloride-responsive alkalosis, it may be necessary to block the effect of aldosterone, e.g. with spironolactone or amiloride. The pH can be corrected rapidly by ventilation using inspired CO_2 and supplemental oxygen to prevent hypoxia.

Respiratory acidosis
This results from a primary decrease in ventilation as a result of depression of the respiratory center, a physical impediment to breathing, such as neurologic or muscular disease, or lung injury.

An acute rise in plasma CO_2 is usually associated with a fall in oxygen levels, dyspnea, reduced consciousness, and eventually coma. Carbon dioxide causes vasodilation which may increase cerebral blood flow, causing headaches and raised intracranial pressure. Systemic vasodilation reduces blood pressure and large rises in plasma CO_2 levels reduce cardiac contractility. In chronic respiratory acidosis, papilledema can occur and there may be reduced bone mineralization as a result of buffering.

Treatment must improve gas exchange. This can be done by treating any underlying disease and by artificial ventilation, or by giving doxapram hydrochloride which triggers central and peripheral chemoreceptors to stimulate ventilation.

Respiratory alkalosis
A primary increase in ventilation can occur as a result of excessive artificial ventilation or in hypoxemia, fever, brain disease, acute cardiopulmonary syndromes, septicemia, liver failure, or pregnancy, and as a side effect of drugs such as salicylates. Plasma bicarbonate falls as a result of reduced bicarbonate reabsorption in the kidney and buffering often includes increased lactate production.

Clinically, there is neuromuscular irritability, with perioral and extremity paresthesia, muscle cramps and tinnitus, hyperreflexia, tetany, and seizures. Cerebral vasoconstriction with reduced blood flow and cardiac dysrhythmias can occur.

Treatment involves correction of the underlying disorder or inhalation of extra CO_2.

Panic attacks with hyperventilation cause transient respiratory alkalosis and are dominated by symptoms of acute hypocalcemia. The alkalosis exposes negative charges on plasma proteins and the free calcium level falls as calcium ions bind to these sites.

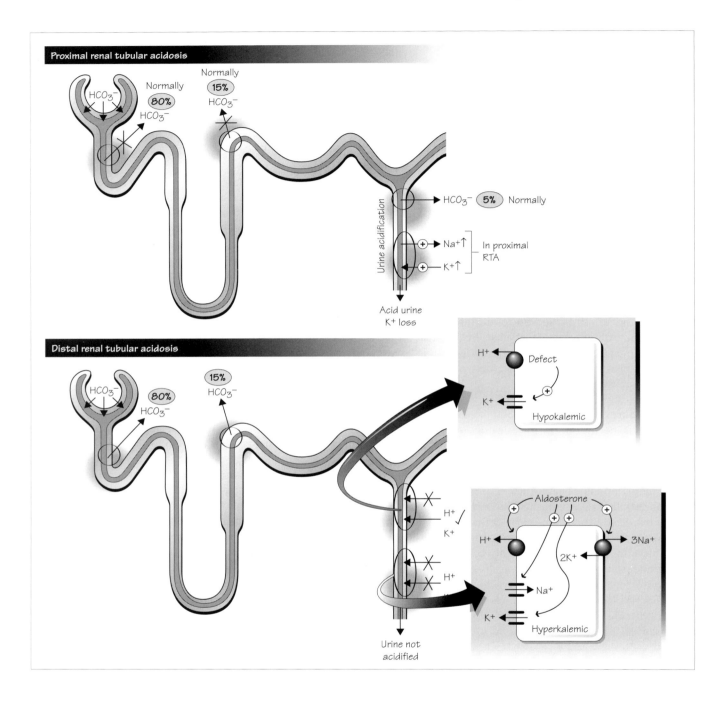

Renal tubular acidosis occurs because the kidney is unable to excrete acid, and hyperchloremic, metabolic acidosis with a normal anion gap occurs (see Chapter 26). Proximal renal tubular acidosis is relatively rare and arises from a defect in proximal tubule bicarbonate reabsorption. It is often associated with other disorders of proximal tubule function. Distal renal tubular acidosis is more common. It produces a more severe acidosis and is associated with many systemic disorders.

Proximal renal tubular acidosis (type II)

Proximal renal tubular acidosis occurs when proximal hydrogen ion secretion and bicarbonate reabsorption fail. In most cases, the specific molecular defects have not been identified, but there is often decreased activity of the Na^+/H^+ exchanger and of the basolateral $Na^+/3HCO_3^-$ co-transporter.

Defects in other proximal tubule functions, such as glucose, phosphate, or urate reabsorption, may be present and this generalized proximal tubular dysfunction is termed Fanconi's syndrome (see Chapter 16). A defect in proximal tubule sodium handling may be responsible because most proximal tubular reabsorption relies to some extent on sodium transport. Causes include generalized damage to the proximal tubule in the context of genetic diseases such as cystinosis or by nephrotoxins such as myeloma light chains.

When proximal bicarbonate reabsorption fails, large amounts of bicarbonate reach the distal tubule. As the capacity of the distal tubule for bicarbonate reabsorption is limited, there is massive bicarbonate loss in the urine, causing acidosis. As a result, the plasma bicarbonate concentration falls and so the concentration of bicarbonate in the filtrate also falls. Eventually the filtrate bicarbonate level falls low enough for it all to be reabsorbed in the distal tubules. At this stage, an acid urine can be excreted and the new low plasma bicarbonate level can be maintained. As a result, a severe acidosis does not occur.

Hypokalemia usually occurs because bicarbonate that is lost takes sodium and water with it. This sodium and water loss can cause volume depletion and triggers aldosterone release. Aldosterone promotes sodium reabsorption in the distal tubule in exchange for potassium. There is often osteomalacia and raised urinary calcium excretion, but urinary citrate levels are high and so stone formation is uncommon.

The diagnosis can be made by showing that the fractional excretion of an administered bicarbonate load is abnormally high when the plasma HCO_3^- level is above 20 mmol/L.

Treatment is with sodium bicarbonate and potassium supplements or potassium-sparing diuretics. Vitamin D and phosphate supplements may be required.

Distal renal tubular acidosis (type I)
In distal renal tubular acidosis, H^+ secretion is impaired in the distal tubule and collecting ducts. In the normal distal tubule urine is made acid and a high H^+ gradient develops. With distal renal tubular acidosis, an acidic urine cannot be produced and a severe metabolic acidosis arises. Typically, the severe acidosis mobilizes bone calcium and causes osteomalacia, nephrocalcinosis, and urinary stone formation. The molecular causes of a number of different types of distal tubular acidosis have been established. The diagnosis can be made by a failure to produce an acid urine even in response to an acid load with NH_4Cl. Distal renal tubular acidosis can be divided according to whether or not there is hyperkalemia.

Hypokalemic distal renal tubular acidosis
In these conditions, potassium handling itself is normal, but potassium is secreted instead of H^+ during sodium reabsorption, causing hypokalemia.

Secretory defects directly reduce H^+ secretion. This arises with deficiency of the H^+ ATPase and less commonly with mutations in the HCO_3^-/Cl^- anion exchanger or deficiency of the cellular carbonic anhydrase. Sjögren's syndrome causes an acquired deficiency of the H^+ ATPase.

Permeability defects caused by toxins such as amphotericin increase the permeability of the distal tubule to H^+, thus preventing a H^+ gradient from developing.

Hyperkalemic distal renal tubular acidosis
In these conditions, there is abnormally reduced potassium and H^+ secretion in the distal tubule. Hyperkalemia worsens the acidosis.

Voltage defects. If distal tubule sodium reabsorption is defective, this reduces the negative luminal charge that promotes both H^+ and K^+ secretion. This can happen with generalized distal tubular damage, including that caused by urinary tract obstruction, interstitial nephritis associated with systemic lupus erythematosus, or amiloride and lithium use.

Hypoaldosteronism. In the distal tubule aldosterone stimulates sodium reabsorption, potassium secretion, and acid secretion by the H^+ ATPase. Without aldosterone, there is sodium wasting, hyperkalemia and acidosis. Low aldosterone levels can result from adrenal failure, inadequate renin secretion, or drugs inhibiting the renin–angiotensin II–aldosterone axis. The most common form is in diabetic nephropathy or tubulointerstitial disease where there is deficient renin production. Cyclosporin A toxicity can have a similar effect.

Treatment of distal renal tubular acidosis involves sodium bicarbonate or sodium citrate administration. Hypokalemia should be corrected with potassium replacement and hyperkalemia can be treated with diuretics. Mineralocorticoid (aldosterone) should be replaced if deficient.

Defective ammoniagenesis
A renal tubular acidosis can arise from inadequate renal ammoniagenesis. When this happens, bicarbonate can be secreted and an acid urine produced, but the amount of acid removed from the body is reduced because the buffering of NH_4^+ is unavailable. The principal causes are hyperkalemia, glucocorticoid deficiency, and loss of renal mass. Hyperkalemia suppresses ammoniagenesis probably by displacing H^+ out of the cells. This causes intracellular alkalosis which opposes cellular loss of the HCO_3^- produced by the ammoniagenesis. Glucocorticoid deficiency suppresses ammoniagenesis because glutamine synthesis, like skeletal muscle protein catabolism, is dependent on glucocorticoids.

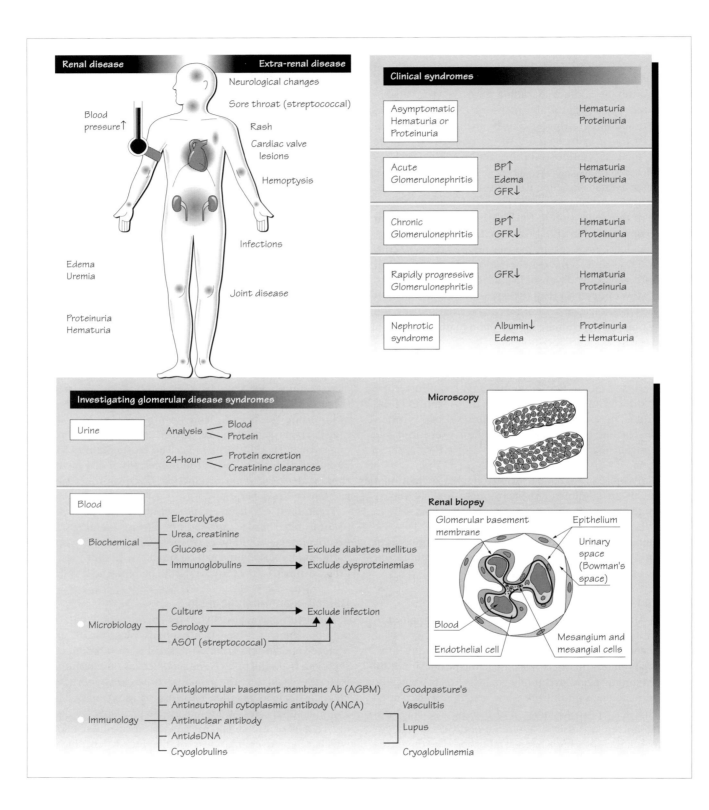

Renal disease

Blood pressure↑

Edema
Uremia

Proteinuria
Hematuria

Extra-renal disease

Neurological changes

Sore throat (streptococcal)

Rash

Cardiac valve lesions

Hemoptysis

Infections

Joint disease

Clinical syndromes

Asymptomatic Hematuria or Proteinuria			Hematuria Proteinuria
Acute Glomerulonephritis		BP↑ Edema GFR↓	Hematuria Proteinuria
Chronic Glomerulonephritis		BP↑ GFR↓	Hematuria Proteinuria
Rapidly progressive Glomerulonephritis		GFR↓	Hematuria Proteinuria
Nephrotic syndrome		Albumin↓ Edema	Proteinuria ± Hematuria

Investigating glomerular disease syndromes

Urine

Analysis ⟨ Blood / Protein

24-hour ⟨ Protein excretion / Creatinine clearances

Microscopy

Blood

● Biochemical ─ Electrolytes
─ Urea, creatinine
─ Glucose ──→ Exclude diabetes mellitus
─ Immunoglobulins ──→ Exclude dysproteinemias

● Microbiology ─ Culture ──→ Exclude infection
─ Serology
─ ASOT (streptococcal)

Renal biopsy

Glomerular basement membrane

Epithelium

Urinary space (Bowman's space)

Blood

Endothelial cell

Mesangium and mesangial cells

● Immunology ─ Antiglomerular basement membrane Ab (AGBM) ── Goodpasture's
─ Antineutrophil cytoplasmic antibody (ANCA) ── Vasculitis
─ Antinuclear antibody
─ AntidsDNA ── Lupus
─ Cryoglobulins ── Cryoglobulinemia

Although many different diseases act on the glomeruli, the effects of glomerular damage are relatively similar whatever the cause.

- **Reduced glomerular filtration** rate resulting from glomerular damage.
- **Proteinuria** caused by protein leakage through the glomerular basement membrane.
- **Hematuria** resulting from active glomerular injury, causing glomerular bleeding.
- **Hypertension** caused by sodium and water retention, often with excess renin secretion.
- **Edema** also resulting from sodium and water retention often with excess renin secretion.

Classification of glomerular disease

Glomerular disease is primary if only the kidney is affected and secondary if the disease process also affects other tissues. Glomerular disease produces the different clinical syndromes discussed below, such as asymptomatic hematuria or the nephrotic syndrome. Glomerular disease can be classified according to the clinical syndrome produced, the histopathologic appearance, or the underlying disease. Only the last is a diagnosis, but the clinical syndrome and histopathologic appearances guide the diagnosis. If the etiology is unknown, the histopathologic description, such as minimal change disease, also serves as the diagnosis, which is really idiopathic minimal change disease.

Pathologic classification

In **proliferative** disease there is abnormal proliferation of cells within the glomerulus. In severe cases, proliferation of cells, especially macrophages within Bowman's capsule, causes an appearance known as a crescent. In **mesangial** disease there is excess production of mesangial matrix. In **membranous** disease, the glomerular basement membrane is damaged and thickened. **Membranoproliferative** disease causes both thickening of the glomerular basement membrane and cellular proliferation, usually of mesangial cells. **Vasculitis** is inflammation of the blood vessels. Usually renal biopsies are interpreted with light microscopy, immunostaining studies, and if necessary electron microscopy.

- *Focal* disease affects only some glomeruli.
- *Diffuse* disease affects all the glomeruli.
- *Segmental* disease affects only part of the glomerulus.
- *Global* disease affects the whole glomerulus.

Clinical syndromes

Glomerular disease produces five major clinical syndromes. These result from different combinations of the possible effects of glomerular injury. **Asymptomatic proteinuria or hematuria** can result from mild glomerular damage. **Acute glomerulonephritis** is the same as **acute nephritic syndrome** and consists of hematuria, an acute fall in glomerular filtration rate (GFR), sodium and water retention, and hyper-tension. **Chronic glomerulonephritis** consists of slow progressive glomerular damage often with proteinuria, hematuria, and hypertension. **Rapidly progressive glomerulonephritis** is a syndrome of very rapid renal failure. There is oliguria and often hematuria and proteinuria, usually without the other features of the nephritic syndrome. **Nephrotic syndrome** consists of heavy proteinuria, leading to hypoalbuminemia and edema (see Chapter 33).

Diagnosing glomerular disease
Clinical assessment

A history of recurrent frank hematuria 1–2 days after an upper respiratory infection suggests IgA nephropathy. Nephritic syndrome occurring 1–3 weeks after an infection suggests postinfective glomerulonephritis, typically post-streptococcal. Hemoptysis with rapidly progressive glomerulonephritis suggests Goodpasture's syndrome. Other features such as skin or joint involvement suggest an underlying condition such as systemic lupus erythematosus. Examination may reveal hypertension, edema, or signs of uremia. It is important to examine for skin, joint, lung, and heart lesions, as well as for neurologic disturbances which can indicate systemic lupus erythematosus, vasculitis, or even infection. Both systemic lupus erythematosus and infective endocarditis can cause cardiac valve lesions and glomerular disease.

Investigations

Analyze urine for blood and protein and examine it with a microscope. Red cell casts indicate active glomerular injury causing glomerular bleeding. Measure serum albumin and quantify any proteinuria with a 24-h urine collection. GFR should be assessed by measuring serum urea and creatinine and, if necessary, creatinine clearance. Selected blood tests may indicate a specific diagnosis.

- Blood glucose, immunoglobulins, and blood cultures may indicate diabetes mellitus, myeloma, or other tumors and infection.
- Significant plasma levels of antiglomerular basement membrane antibody indicate antiglomerular basement membrane (Goodpasture's) disease.
- Significant levels of antineutrophil cytoplasmic antibodies (ANCA) suggest systemic vasculitis.
- Antinuclear antibodies with specificity for double-stranded DNA and low complement levels indicate systemic lupus erythematosus.
- Cryoglobulins are present in cryoglobulinemia.
- Lung function tests may be abnormal if there is pulmonary hemorrhage (Goodpasture's syndrome) because blood in the alveoli absorbs the carbon monoxide used to measure gas transfer, which spuriously raises the gas transfer coefficient.

Unless the diagnosis is clinically obvious, renal biopsy is performed.

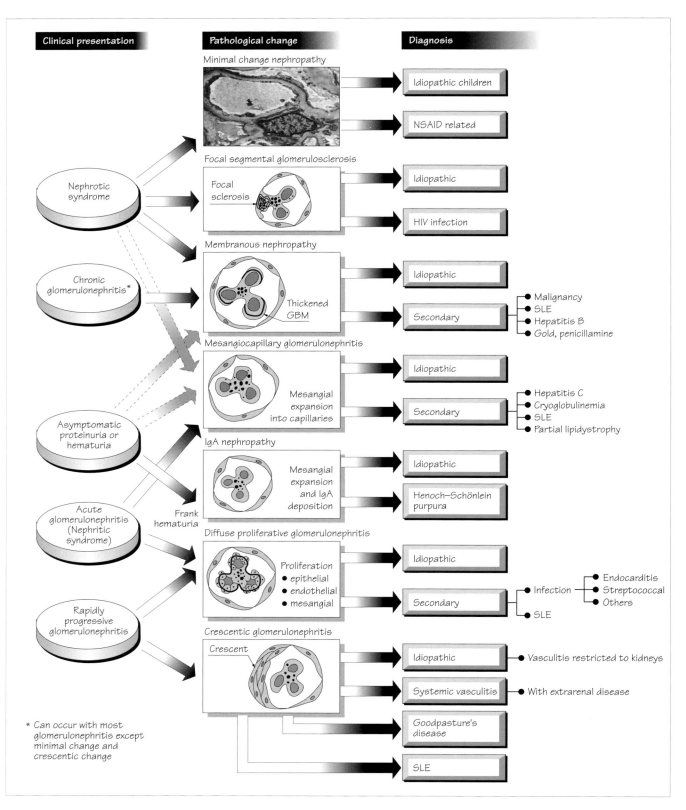

Diseases of the glomerular basement membrane

Minimal change nephropathy

Minimal change nephropathy accounts for 90% of the nephrotic syndrome in children and 20% in adults. In children, it is associated with atopy (asthma, eczema, and hay fever) and it often follows an upper respiratory tract infection. The disease is termed 'minimal change nephropathy,' because light microscopy and immunostaining is normal. However, electron microscopy shows fusion of the podocyte foot processes. The condition responds to steroids and, if it relapses, cyclosporin is useful. Renal impairment does not occur. Non-steroidal anti-inflammatory drugs can cause minimal change disease.

Focal segmental glomerulosclerosis

This accounts for 15% of the adult nephrotic syndrome and can also cause hematuria and hypertension. Focal and segmental scarring is seen, and the scars contain immunoglobulins and complement. Electron microscopy shows podocyte foot process fusion as in minimal change nephropathy. The two conditions may be different results of an essentially similar disease process. Some patients respond to steroids and relapse is reduced by cyclosporin or cyclophosphamide. Many patients eventually develop end-stage renal failure and the disease can recur after renal transplantation. A variant is associated with HIV infection.

Membranous nephropathy

Membranous nephropathy is the most common cause of the nephrotic syndrome in older patients. There is proteinuria and often renal impairment. Histologically, there is thickening of the glomerular basement membrane. It is usually idiopathic, but can be secondary to malignancy, hepatitis B, systemic lupus erythematosus, or use of gold or penicillamine drugs. Some patients respond to steroids and chlorambucil or cyclophosphamide, but a minority develop end-stage renal disease.

Proliferative glomerulopathy

Mesangiocapillary glomerulonephritis

This is also known as membranoproliferative glomerulonephritis. It is uncommon and occurs mainly in young adults and children. The presentation varies from asymptomatic hematuria or proteinuria to the usual presentation with combined nephrotic and nephritic syndromes. Most patients develop end-stage renal failure and there is no useful treatment. There is mesangial cell proliferation, excess mesangial matrix, and thickening of the glomerular basement membrane. Most cases are of type I with subendothelial and mesangial immune deposits. In the rarer type II disease, there are immune deposits in the membrane. Type I disease is usually associated with systemic lupus erythematosus, infection, or cryoglobulinemia. Patients have low levels of C3 and C4 as a result of complement depletion. Type II disease is associated with antibodies that activate and deplete complement, and some patients have the rare disorder partial lipodystrophy.

IgA nephropathy (Berger's disease)

Worldwide this is the most common primary glomerular disease. The typical presentation is in a young man who develops macroscopic hematuria 1–2 days after an upper respiratory tract infection. It can also present with asymptomatic microscopic hematuria, proteinuria, and renal impairment. There is mesangial cell proliferation, increased mesangial matrix, and IgA deposition in the mesangium. Patients often have raised serum IgA levels. Treatment is usually unsuccessful. Nearly a third of patients eventually develop end-stage renal disease and recurrence can occur after renal transplantation.

Henoch–Schönlein purpura

This disease mainly affects children aged under 10. Typically, there is a purpuric rash on the ankles, buttocks, and elbows, abdominal pain, and renal disease. There is usually hematuria, proteinuria, hypertension, fluid retention, and renal impairment, sometimes with the nephrotic syndrome. The histology looks the same as IgA nephropathy. Most children recover fully without treatment.

Diffuse proliferative glomerulonephritis (diffuse endocapillary proliferative glomerulonephritis)

This pathologic appearance is typical of post-streptococcal glomerulonephritis, but it can follow other infections, especially infective endocarditis. The classic presentation is nephritic syndrome occurring several weeks after infection. Most patients have low complement levels. There is endothelial and mesangial cell proliferation and glomerular infiltration by neutrophils and monocytes. There is deposition of complement, IgM, and IgG on the basement membrane and in the mesangium. Electron microscopy shows subepithelial deposits. Antibiotics are given to eradicate any lingering infection and only a few percent of patients develop end-stage renal disease.

Crescentic glomerulonephritis

Crescents are accumulations of macrophages within Bowman's capsule and indicate severe glomerular injury. There are many causes, especially antiglomerular basement membrane disease (Goodpasture's syndrome), systemic vasculitis, and systemic lupus erythematosus, IgA nephropathy, Henoch–Schönlein disease, vasculitis, and cryoglobulinemia. 'Idiopathic rapidly progressive glomerulonephritis,' may be a form of limited vasculitis.

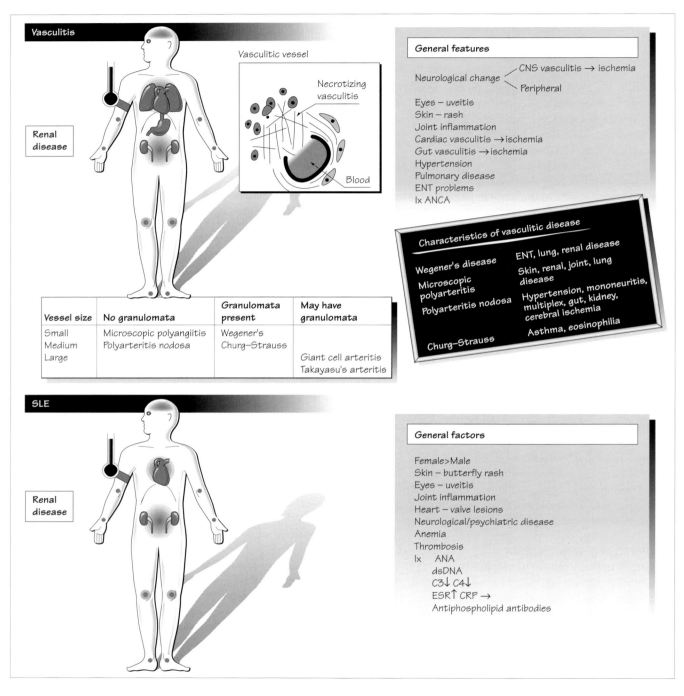

Vasculitis

Vasculitic vessel

Necrotizing vasculitis

Blood

Renal disease

General features

Neurological change
— CNS vasculitis → ischemia
— Peripheral

Eyes – uveitis
Skin – rash
Joint inflammation
Cardiac vasculitis → ischemia
Gut vasculitis → ischemia
Hypertension
Pulmonary disease
ENT problems
Ix ANCA

Characteristics of vasculitic disease

Wegener's disease	ENT, lung, renal disease
Microscopic polyarteritis	Skin, renal, joint, lung disease
Polyarteritis nodosa	Hypertension, mononeuritis, multiplex, gut, kidney, cerebral ischemia
Churg–Strauss	Asthma, eosinophilia

Vessel size	No granulomata	Granulomata present	May have granulomata
Small Medium Large	Microscopic polyangiitis Polyarteritis nodosa	Wegener's Churg–Strauss	Giant cell arteritis Takayasu's arteritis

SLE

Renal disease

General factors

Female>Male
Skin – butterfly rash
Eyes – uveitis
Joint inflammation
Heart – valve lesions
Neurological/psychiatric disease
Anemia
Thrombosis
Ix   ANA
       dsDNA
       C3↓ C4↓
       ESR↑ CRP →
       Antiphospholipid antibodies

Antiglomerular basement membrane disease (Goodpasture's syndrome)

This disease is caused by antibodies against the C-terminal end of the α_3 chain of type IV collagen in the glomerular basement membrane and the alveolar basement membrane in the lung. The antibody binds to these membranes trigger-ing inflammation. This causes rapidly progressive crescentic glomerulonephritis with *acute renal failure* and *lung hemorrhage*. Patients are usually male with the tissue type HLA-DR2. If untreated, patients die from pulmonary hemorrhage or renal failure. Treatment involves plasma exchange to remove the antibodies and immunosuppression with steroids and cyclophosphamide to inhibit glomerular inflammation and reduce antibody production. If treated early most patients recover and relapse is uncommon.

Primary systemic vasculitis

The primary vasculitic diseases produce necrotizing inflammation of vessels and often affect the kidneys, respiratory tract, joints, skin, and nervous system. They are classified according to the size of the vessels affected and the presence or absence of granulomata (see figure). The two small vessel diseases (and less commonly Churg–Strauss syndrome) can cause a focal segmental proliferative glomerulonephritis with necrosis and crescent formation. Clinically, they often present as rapidly progressive glomerulonephritis. Histologically, there is infiltration of the glomeruli by neutrophils, but no complement or immunoglobulin deposition. Antineutrophil cytoplasmic antibodies (ANCA) against neutrophil granule contents are usually present. Patients with Wegener's granulomatosis have a cytoplasmic or c-ANCA reactivity against proteinase 3. Patients with microscopic polyangiitis have a perinuclear or p-ANCA reactivity against myeloperoxidase. Therapy is initially with steroids and cyclophosphamide. After several months, azathioprine is substituted for the cyclophosphamide. Plasma exchange is sometimes used in the acute phase. **Idiopathic rapidly progressive glomerulonephritis** is a small vessel vasculitis affecting only the kidney. There is no ANCA, but it is treated like the other small vessel disorders.

Systemic lupus erythematosus

This is a multisystem disease which can affect the nervous system, joints, skin, kidneys, and heart. The renal effects vary and have been classified by the World Health Organization as: type I—minimal change; type II—mesangial; type III—focal proliferative; type IV—diffuse proliferative; and type V—membranous. The renal presentation depends on the histologic lesion. It is typically nephrotic syndrome or renal impairment and can be acute. There are usually antinuclear antibodies to double-stranded DNA and low complement levels. Typically the ESR (erythrocyte sedimentation rate) is raised, but the CRP (C-reactive protein) is normal unless there is infection. Treatment for renal disease with steroids and cyclophosphamide or azathioprine is usually helpful.

Cryoglobulinemia

Cryoglobulins are immunoglobulins that precipitate in the cold. They occur in inflammatory or neoplastic diseases including myeloma, lymphoma, multisystem autoimmune diseases, and chronic infection. Plasma complement levels are usually low. Typically, cryoglobulins cause a type I mesangiocapillary glomerulonephritis. Mixed essential cryoglobulinemia is usually caused by hepatitis C infection.

The clinical presentation is usually of a purpuric vasculitic rash, arthralgia, peripheral neuropathy, and glomerulonephritis. Cryoglobulins are removed by plasma exchange in severe disease.

Dysproteinemias

These disorders are characterized by excess antibody production by benign or malignant plasma cell activity. Malignant disease or myeloma can cause various renal problems, including glomerular deposition of amyloid fibrils, tubular toxicity from filtered light chains, and mesangiocapillary glomerulonephritis resulting from glomerular deposition of light chains.

Rheumatoid arthritis and connective tissue diseases

Rheumatoid arthritis can cause renal amyloid deposition, mesangial proliferative glomerulonephritis, membranous nephropathy, or a focal segmental glomerulonephritis with vasculitis and necrosis. Systemic sclerosis or scleroderma is rarely associated with a crescentic glomerulonephritis. More commonly, there is hyperplasia of small renal arteries. Any additional vasospasm causes acute renal ischemia. This 'renal crisis' triggers renin release which worsens the vasospasm and promotes severe hypertension.

Amyloidosis

Amyloid protein is a combination of amyloid P protein with either antibody light chains (*AL amyloid*) or the inflammatory amyloid A protein (*AA amyloid*). AL amyloid is typical of dysproteinemias, whereas AA amyloid is typical of chronic inflammatory diseases. Amyloid deposition can damage the kidney, liver, spleen, heart, tongue, and nervous system. Amyloidosis can cause proteinuria and a nephrotic syndrome. Histologically, amyloid can be visualized by Congo red staining in the glomeruli, the tubules, and the blood vessels. Treatment aims to reduce production of the amyloid proteins by treating any underlying dysproteinemia or inflammatory disease.

Drug causes of glomerular disease

Gold and penicillamine can both cause membranous nephropathy. Hydralazine causes a lupus-like disease. Non-steroidal anti-inflammatory drugs can cause minimal change glomerular disease, with nephrotic syndrome and often with an interstitial nephritis.

Hereditary and other causes of glomerular disease

Thin basement membrane disease causes asymptomatic microscopic hematuria. The condition is inherited and does not normally cause renal deterioration. Alport's disease is usually an X-linked mutation in the α_5 chain of type IV collagen, a component of the glomerular basement membrane. It causes proteinuria, hematuria, renal failure, and sensorineural deafness.

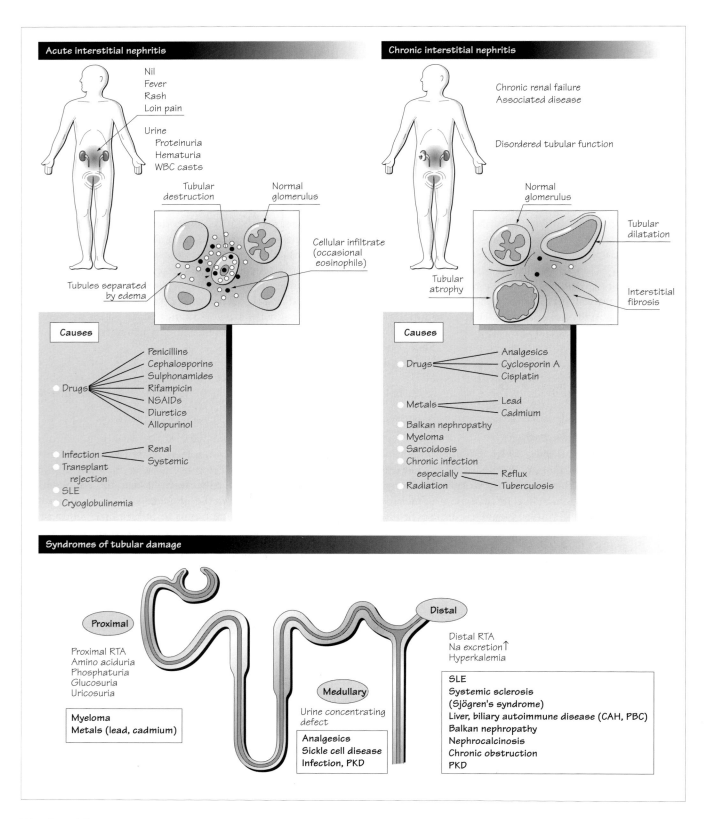

Acute interstitial nephritis

Nil
Fever
Rash
Loin pain

Urine
  Proteinuria
  Hematuria
  WBC casts

Tubular destruction

Normal glomerulus

Cellular infiltrate (occasional eosinophils)

Tubules separated by edema

Causes

Drugs
- Penicillins
- Cephalosporins
- Sulphonamides
- Rifampicin
- NSAIDs
- Diuretics
- Allopurinol

Infection — Renal / Systemic
Transplant rejection
SLE
Cryoglobulinemia

Chronic interstitial nephritis

Chronic renal failure
Associated disease

Disordered tubular function

Normal glomerulus

Tubular dilatation

Tubular atrophy

Interstitial fibrosis

Causes

Drugs
- Analgesics
- Cyclosporin A
- Cisplatin

Metals
- Lead
- Cadmium

Balkan nephropathy
Myeloma
Sarcoidosis
Chronic infection
  especially — Reflux / Tuberculosis
Radiation

Syndromes of tubular damage

Proximal

Proximal RTA
Amino aciduria
Phosphaturia
Glucosuria
Uricosuria

Myeloma
Metals (lead, cadmium)

Medullary

Urine concentrating defect

Analgesics
Sickle cell disease
Infection, PKD

Distal

Distal RTA
Na excretion↑
Hyperkalemia

SLE
Systemic sclerosis
(Sjögren's syndrome)
Liver, biliary autoimmune disease (CAH, PBC)
Balkan nephropathy
Nephrocalcinosis
Chronic obstruction
PKD

The tubules and the renal interstitium are in intimate contact and are both affected by a range of disease processes. The clinical presentation is determined by the effect on tubular function. Typically, the tubules either become blocked, which reduces glomerular filtration, or their transport functions become impaired, which reduces water and solute reabsorption. Important presentations of tubulointerstitial damage are acute and chronic interstitial nephritis. Interstitial changes also occur in acute tubular necrosis, acute renal transplant rejection, and urinary tract obstruction. Certain diseases, mainly hereditary, impair tubular function without causing interstitial changes.

Acute interstitial nephritis

This causes acute diffuse renal inflammation and there can be a rapid deterioration in renal function. Acute interstitial nephritis is usually asymptomatic but, if it is drug induced, there may be a maculopapular rash, fever, or eosinophilia. Lumbar pain can occur, probably as a result of stretching of the renal capsule. There may be mild proteinuria, microscopic hematuria, white blood cell casts, and eosinophils in the urine. Ultrasonography usually shows slightly enlarged kidneys. Formal diagnosis requires a renal biopsy. There is infiltration of the interstitium with inflammatory cells, particularly monocytes and T cells. The tubular basement membrane may be disrupted and tubules may be compressed by the infiltrating cells. Treatment involves discontinuation of any drug that could be the cause, treatment of any infection, and often immunosuppression with steroids. The prognosis is good.

Etiology of acute interstitial nephritis

The main cause is an allergic reaction to a drug, particularly *non-steroidal anti-inflammatory drugs (NSAIDs), diuretics, and antibiotics* (especially penicillins, cephalosporins, rifampin (rifampicin), and sulfonamides). Systemic or renal infection, typically acute pyelonephritis, can cause an acute interstitial nephritis. Gout causes excess urate excretion and urate crystals can precipitate in the tubules causing tubular obstruction and triggering inflammation.

Chronic interstitial nephritis

Typically, this presents as either chronic renal failure or with symptoms of an associated primary disease. Hypertension is common, the glomerular filtration rate (GFR) is reduced, and there is mild proteinuria, microscopic hematuria, and inflammatory cells in the urine. Tubular transport and reabsorption can be impaired, resulting in features such as glycosuria. Destruction of interstitial erythropoietin-producing cells can cause anemia. Tubular cells are flat and atrophic, the tubules are dilated, and there is interstitial fibrosis with a mononuclear cell infiltrate.

Etiology of chronic interstitial nephritis

Antibody light chains are filtered in the glomerulus and normally reabsorbed in the proximal tubule by receptor-mediated endocytosis. In **myeloma**, the high level of light chains saturates this reabsorption leading to light chain excretion (Bence Jones proteinuria). Light chains are toxic to tubules and cause tubular inflammation and damage. Excess use of **analgesics** such as aspirin, paracetamol (acetaminophen), NSAIDs (and in the past, phenacetin) causes chronic interstitial nephritis and sometimes papillary necrosis. **Other causes** of chronic interstitial nephritis include excess lead or cadmium intake, radiation, sarcoidosis, and Balkan nephropathy (an endemic chronic interstitial disease affecting countries around the Balkan sea).

Papillary necrosis

The medulla receives all its blood supply from the vasa recta which makes the papillae highly vulnerable to ischemic damage and hypoxia. In addition, the counter-current system concentrates some toxins, such as analgesics, in the medulla and papillae. If there is severe medullary ischemia or interstitial damage, the function of the loop of Henle and collecting ducts may be impaired. In the worst cases, damaged papillae can slough off and even obstruct the ureters. Causes include analgesic use, diabetes mellitus, infection, and sickle-cell disease. In sickle-cell disease, medullary ischemia promotes red blood cell sickling in the papillae. In diabetes mellitus, infection and vascular disease promote ischemic papillary damage.

Disorders of tubular function

Disorders of tubular function include aminoacidurias, renal tubular acidoses, Bartter's syndrome, vitamin D-resistant rickets, nephrogenic diabetes insipidus, and Fanconi's syndrome (see Chapters 16, 18, 24, 28). There are three main patterns of tubular damage which reflect the transport functions of the damaged tubule segment. The abnormalities of tubular function can occur alone in specific diseases or as part of acute or more usually chronic tubulointerstitial nephritis.

Proximal tubule damage impairs proximal tubular reabsorption. Possible consequences include aminoaciduria, glycosuria, phosphaturia, uricosuria, and bicarbonaturia leading to metabolic acidosis (proximal renal tubular acidosis).

Distal tubule damage can impair distal bicarbonate reabsorption and aldosterone-regulated sodium reabsorption, and the related potassium secretion. The bicarbonaturia causes metabolic acidosis (distal renal tubular acidosis).

Medullary damage affects the loop of Henle and collecting ducts, reducing the kidneys' ability to concentrate urine. This can occur after infection, analgesic use, and sickle-cell disease, and in the polyuric recovery phase of acute tubular necrosis.

33 Proteinuria and the nephrotic syndrome

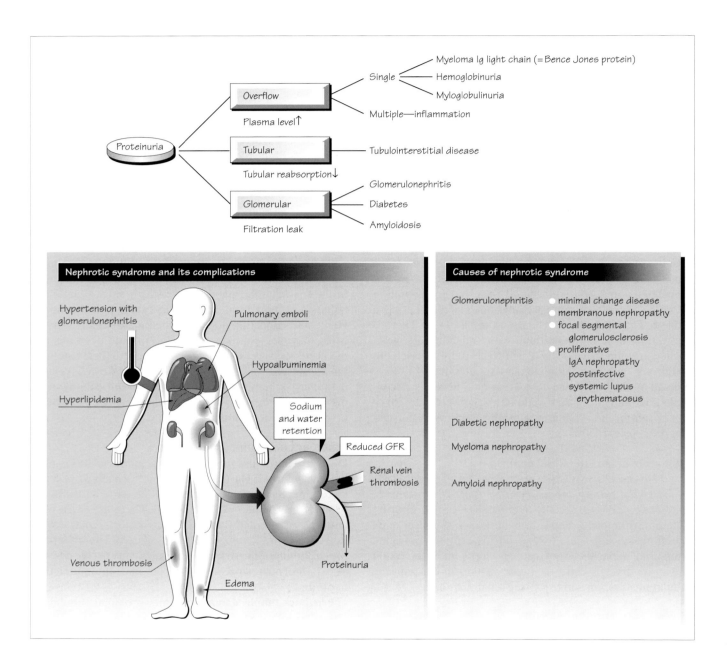

Clinically detectable proteinuria is abnormal and is usually an early marker of renal disease. The nephrotic syndrome occurs when proteinuria is severe enough to cause hypoalbuminemia and there is associated sodium and water retention, causing edema. All causes of nephrotic proteinuria result in abnormal foot processes consistent with defects in the slit diaphragm and the size selectivity of filtration.

Types of proteinuria

Plasma proteins are filtered at the glomerulus according to their size and charge. Small proteins of less than 20 kDa are freely filtered, then reabsorbed, and degraded in the proximal tubule. This process catabolizes hormones, such as insulin, and small immunologic molecules, such as immunoglobulin light chains. Therefore, isolated loss of small proteins in the urine (**selective proteinuria**) indicates either *overflow proteinuria* (caused by excess serum and filtered protein levels overwhelming normal tubular reabsorption), or *tubular proteinuria* (resulting from impaired tubular reabsorption). The filtration barrier is normal. Large proteins such as albumin, transferrin, and IgG are not normally filtered and are only lost in urine if the glomerular filtration barrier is damaged. This relatively **non-selective proteinuria** is termed *glomerular proteinuria*.

Proteinuria is detected with urine dipsticks and can be quantified with a 24-h urine collection. Proteinuria in the nephrotic range is >3.5 g/24 h. A high urine protein : creatinine ratio above 3.5 (g/g) also signifies nephrotic range proteinuria. Very sensitive radioimmunoassays are used to detect very low levels of albuminuria in early diabetic nephropathy. **Urinary protein electrophoresis** can distinguish different types of proteinuria. With tubular and overflow proteinuria, only low molecular weight proteins are present. With overflow proteinuria, there is generally one abundant protein in the urine, typically an immunoglobulin light chain resulting from a B-cell disorder such as myeloma. Rarely, inflammation can cause overflow of many small acute phase proteins. Glomerular proteinuria is dominated by albumin because of its high plasma concentration and lesser amounts of transferrin and IgG.

Clinical features of nephrotic syndrome

Nephrotic patients usually present with edema. Their urine may be frothy because of its high protein content. The most common causes are minimal change glomerulonephritis in children and membranous nephropathy or focal segmental glomerulosclerosis in adults (see Chapter 30). A prothrombotic state, hypertension, and hyperlipidemia all contribute to a higher incidence of ischemic heart disease in nephrotic patients. Unless there is obvious diabetic nephropathy or clinically typical childhood minimal change glomerulonephritis, a histologic diagnosis is made by renal biopsy.

Renal sodium retention and edema

Hypoalbuminemia may reduce intravascular volume leading to renal hypoperfusion and renin-mediated hyperaldosteronism (see Chapter 20).

Protein loss, malnutrition, and infection

Urinary protein loss can cause negative protein balance and protein malnutrition. Patients have a tendency to infection, possibly because IgG and other immune proteins are lost in the urine. Pneumococcal infection was a particular problem, but the use of pneumococcal vaccine and prophylactic antibiotics have reduced this.

Thrombosis

Thromboregulatory proteins, such as antithrombin III, protein S, and protein C, are lost in the urine and hypopro-teinemia increases liver synthesis of fibrinogen, raising fibrinogen levels. These changes promote venous thrombosis, especially in the renal and deep leg veins. Pulmonary emboli can then occur. Renal vein thrombosis can cause a sudden deterioration in renal function with flank pain and hematuria.

Hyperlipidemia

There is increased hepatic lipid and apolipoprotein synthesis and reduced chylomicron and very-low-density lipoprotein (VLDL) catabolism. These changes may result from loss in the urine of liporegulatory substances and cause a rise in plasma LDL-cholesterol and VLDL. Hyperlipidemia requires diet and drug therapy.

Renal impairment

Glomerular filtration is often reduced and nephrotic kidneys are vulnerable to pre-renal acute renal failure. Disruption of the normal arrangement of epithelial foot processes probably reduces the number of functional interpodocyte filtration slits. Although each slit is highly permeable, there may be a reduction in the total surface area for filtration and so a fall in glomerular filtration rate (GFR).

Treatment

Any underlying disease process should be treated. Some general measures may also be useful. Angiotensin-converting enzyme (ACE) inhibitors often reduce proteinuria, possibly by a direct effect on the filtration barrier. Non-steroidal anti-inflammatory drugs such as indomethacin reduce GFR, filtration fraction, and proteinuria but can worsen sodium retention and trigger acute renal failure. Both ACE inhibitors and non-steroidal anti-inflammatory drugs can cause hyperkalemia. In extreme cases, renal embolization or nephrectomy has been performed to prevent severe proteinuria. Edema can be treated with sodium restriction and diuretics (see Chapter 20). Prophylactic support stockings and heparin or warfarin can help to prevent thrombosis with severe proteinuria or hypoalbuminemia.

Pregnancy and proteinuria

Most causes of proteinuria can also occur during pregnancy, especially renal disease caused by systemic lupus erythematosus. However, in the last trimester of pregnancy, *pre-eclampsia can cause hypertension, edema, and proteinuria*. If protein loss is high, nephrotic syndrome can result. Pre-eclampsia may result from abnormal endothelial function and aberrant prostaglandin synthesis triggered by the presence of the fetus. In high-risk individuals, low-dose aspirin provides some prophylaxis. Treatment is bed rest, anti-hypertensive therapy, and early delivery if the condition worsens. Untreated it can result in seizures and death.

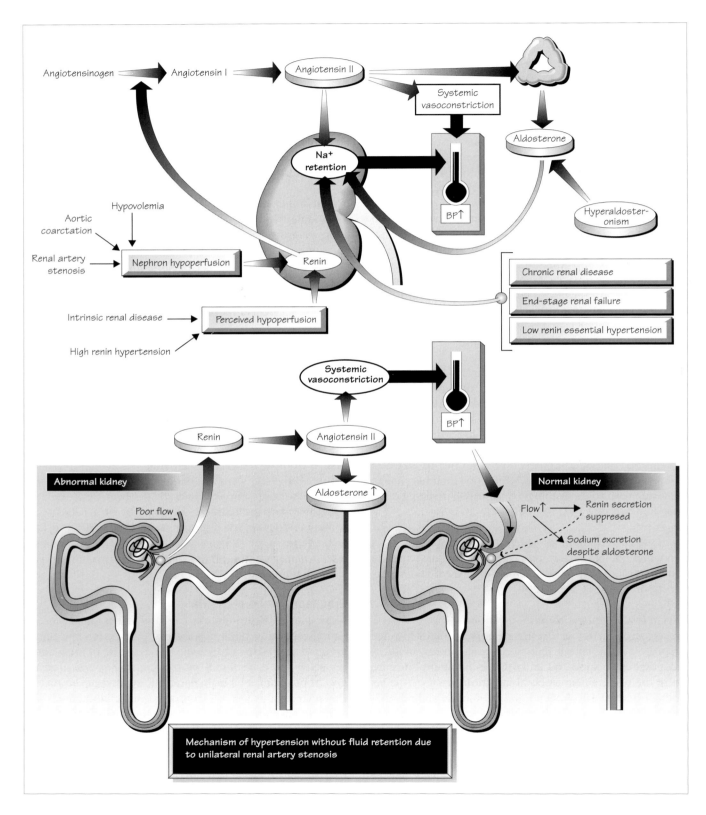

Hypertension is defined as blood pressure greater than 140/90 mmHg. It can damage vessels and organs and increases mortality. Treatment improves the prognosis. If a cause is identified, hypertension is said to be secondary; if there is no identifiable cause, it is termed primary or essential hypertension. Blood pressure is determined by cardiac output, systemic vascular resistance, and circulatory volume. The key determinant of systemic vascular resistance is vasoconstriction of arterioles and the key determinant of circulatory volume is renal sodium handling.

Causes of secondary hypertension
Renal artery stenosis
Renal artery stenosis (see Chapter 37) reduces renal blood flow and the glomerular filtration rate (GFR), stimulating renin release and angiotensin II production. Angiotensin II causes hypertension by vasoconstriction and stimulation of aldosterone release and sodium retention. If both kidneys are affected, the hypervolemia and hypertension eventually restore renal perfusion and renin levels fall slightly. If only one kidney is normal, the hypertension increases its GFR. This promotes sodium excretion by the healthy kidney, but the stenosed kidney remains underperfused and continues to produce very high renin levels.

Primary hyperaldosteronism
Primary hyperaldosteronism accounts for 1–2% of all hypertension. Excess aldosterone increases renal sodium retention and potassium secretion. The resulting hypervolemia causes hypertension. Renin production is suppressed because renal perfusion pressure and sodium chloride delivery to the macula densa are increased.

Intrinsic renal disease
Any renal disease can cause hypertension. *Severe renal impairment* reduces sodium excretion and causes hypervolemia and hypertension which is 'salt sensitive,' because it is increased by salt intake. With *milder renal impairment*, perceived renal hypoperfusion promotes renin secretion and angiotensin II-mediated vasoconstriction. This hypertension is not salt sensitive and is termed *salt resistant*.

Other causes of hypertension
Coarctation of the aorta reduces renal perfusion and triggers renin secretion. Characteristically, pulses are weaker in the legs than in the arms. **Steroids** cause sodium retention and hypertension. This is a mineralocorticoid effect of administered and endogenous glucocorticoids. **Catecholamine** release by a pheochromocytoma causes vasoconstrictive hypertension. **Drugs** can cause hypertension, especially steroids, cyclosporin, and estrogens in oral contraceptives.

Pathogenesis of primary hypertension
Essential hypertension is characterized by an increase in peripheral resistance. This can be caused by two mechanisms which may coexist.

High-renin/salt-resistant/dry essential hypertension
These patients have a raised renin level for their body sodium content. This causes angiotensin II release with vasoconstriction, aldosterone secretion, and sodium retention. However, the filtration fraction and sodium excretion increase to a greater extent and the patient can become hypovolemic. The hypertension is salt resistant because salt excretion is not impaired. The excess angiotensin II causes vasoconstriction and also promotes vascular smooth muscle hypertrophy and proliferation. High renin and angiotensin II levels in hypertension correlate with vascular and end-organ damage. Mild hypovolemia may cause mild tissue ischemia. High renin hypertension responds best to inhibition of the renin–angiotensin II axis with **angiotensin-converting enzyme inhibitors, angiotensin II antagonists**, or β **blockers** (which inhibit renin secretion).

Low-renin/salt-sensitive/wet essential hypertension
These patients have renal sodium and water retention which suppress renin secretion. The hypertension worsens with a high salt intake. Sodium retention may be caused by increased sympathetic adrenergic activity or a defect in sodium-coupled calcium transport. Excess sodium may cause vasoconstriction by altering smooth muscle calcium fluxes. Patients respond to **sodium restriction**, **diuretics**, α_1-**adrenergic blockers**, and **calcium channel antagonists**.

Clinical evaluation of hypertension
Hypertension is diagnosed if blood pressure is raised on three separate occasions or on 24-h ambulatory blood pressure monitoring. A large cuff must be used with a large arm, otherwise a falsely high reading will be obtained. The beginning of the first sound indicates the systolic pressure and the end of the last sound the diastolic pressure. Hypertensive retinopathy confirms the presence of hypertension and may indicate malignant hypertension. Hypertension is often associated with obesity, excess alcohol intake, insulin resistance, and gout. *Baseline investigations* include urinalysis, a full blood count, serum electrolytes, glucose and uric acid, and electrocardiography (ECG), ideally with echocardiography to identify left ventricular hypertrophy. Hypokalemia suggests primary hyperaldosteronism. Further investigations may include plasma and urinary vanillylmandelic acid (VMA) levels to exclude pheochromocytomas, adrenal function tests to check for steroid excess, and renal angiography to exclude renal artery stenosis.

35 Hypertension: complications and therapy

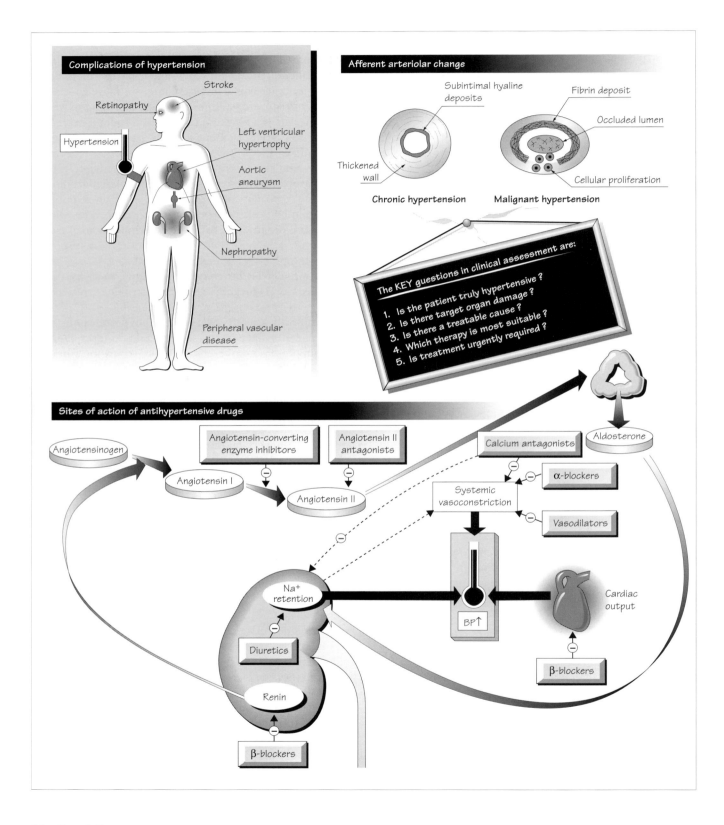

Complications of hypertension

Stroke
Retinopathy
Hypertension
Left ventricular hypertrophy
Aortic aneurysm
Nephropathy
Peripheral vascular disease

Afferent arteriolar change

Subintimal hyaline deposits
Fibrin deposit
Occluded lumen
Thickened wall
Cellular proliferation

Chronic hypertension
Malignant hypertension

The KEY questions in clinical assessment are:
1. Is the patient truly hypertensive ?
2. Is there target organ damage ?
3. Is there a treatable cause ?
4. Which therapy is most suitable ?
5. Is treatment urgently required ?

Sites of action of antihypertensive drugs

Angiotensinogen
Angiotensin-converting enzyme inhibitors
Angiotensin II antagonists
Calcium antagonists
Aldosterone
Angiotensin I
Angiotensin II
α-blockers
Systemic vasoconstriction
Vasodilators
Na⁺ retention
BP↑
Cardiac output
Diuretics
β-blockers
Renin
β-blockers

Complications of hypertension

Renal complications

Microalbuminuria and dipstick proteinuria are early signs of hypertensive nephropathy. Blood pressure control slows the rate of renal damage. The groups most likely to develop hypertensive renal damage are elderly people, obese individuals, black patients, and those from the Indian subcontinent, especially those with diabetes. The primary insult is damage to the renal vessels from the raised pressure. In the interlobular artery walls, muscle is replaced by sclerotic tissue. The afferent arteriole walls undergo hyalinization—the subintimal deposition of lipids and glycoproteins exuded from plasma. Damage to these resistance vessels exposes the glomerular capillary endothelium to hypertension. This reduces glomerular blood flow and filtration, and promotes proteinuria. Inflammatory proteins are exuded from the plasma and ultimately there is glomerular sclerosis or ischemic atrophy.

Cardiovascular complications

The high vascular resistance strains the heart causing left ventricular hypertrophy. Hypertension also increases the atherosclerosis of arteries.

Retinopathy

Retinopathy is common and is graded according to severity. Grade 3 or 4 indicates accelerated or 'malignant' hypertension. **Grade 1**—Arterial spasm, tortuous arteries, silver-wire appearance. **Grade 2**—Arteriovenous nipping. Veins appear narrowed as arteries pass over them. **Grade 3**—Hemorrhage, including flame hemorrhage. Lipid extravasation causes exudates; hard exudates are old, but soft exudates or cotton-wool spots indicate acute severe hypertension. **Grade 4**—Papilledema. A swollen optic disc.

Malignant or accelerated hypertension

This is severe hypertension with grade 3 or 4 retinal changes and renal damage. It can arise anew or as a complication of essential or secondary hypertension. The central feature is renal vessel damage, usually caused by hypertension. This damage reduces renal blood flow, triggering renin secretion, which promotes further hypertension and sodium retention. Damage to the endothelium can cause fibrinoid necrosis—fibrin enters the vessel wall, triggering cellular proliferation, vessel occlusion, and ischemia.

The clinical presentation can be of headache, visual disturbance, or shortness of breath as a result of cardiac problems. Renal impairment is common, often with hematuria and proteinuria. Damaged vessels can harm red blood cells, causing a microangiopathic hemolytic anemia. **Treatment** is with angiotensin-converting enzyme (ACE) inhibitors, angiotensin antagonists, or β blockers to block the renin cycle. Care is required because patients may have renal artery stenosis (see Chapter 37). Diuretics promote sodium excretion. Hypertensive encephalopathy, pulmonary edema, or severe acute renal disease may require intravenous treatment with sodium nitroprusside, hydralazine, labetalol, or a nitrate preparation.

Treatment of hypertension

Unless there is severe hypertension, end-organ damage, or malignant hypertension, treatment is not urgent. Blood pressure may be improved by exercise, reduced alcohol consumption, and correction of obesity. A reduction in salt intake will help salt-sensitive hypertension, especially if there is renal impairment (see Chapter 34).

• **β Blockers** suppress renin secretion, reduce cardiac output, and may have a centrally mediated effect. Lowering the cardiac output can worsen the symptoms of peripheral vascular disease. β Blockers blunt the catecholaminergic effects that normally warn people with diabetes of hypoglycemia. β_1-Selective blockers avoid the bronchospasm of β_2 blockade.

• **ACE inhibitors** inhibit angiotensin II production. They reduce intraglomerular pressure by dilating efferent arterioles more than afferent arterioles. This reduces proteinuria and glomerulosclerosis. Complications include hyperkalemia caused by reduced aldosterone production and renal impairment if renal artery stenosis is present. ACE degrades bradykinin, so ACE inhibitors cause high bradykinin levels that can cause a cough.

• **Angiotensin II receptor antagonists,** such as losartan, have the same effect as ACE inhibitors. Cough is not a problem.

• **Calcium channel blockers** cause vasodilation. In salt-sensitive hypertension, they also increase sodium excretion by poorly understood mechanisms. Verapamil and diltiazem reduce atrioventricular nodal conduction and should not be given with β blockers. Nifedipine dilates only afferent arterioles, allowing systemic hypertension to cause intraglomerular hypertension.

• **Diuretics,** mainly thiazides, are used in hypertension, but these are ineffective if the glomerular filtration rate is low. Furosemide may then be beneficial.

• α_1-**Antagonists,** such as doxazosin, block catecholaminergic vasoconstriction and can cause postural hypotension. However, they improve insulin sensitivity, lipid profiles, and sometimes erectile function, and can increase urine flow rates when there is prostatic hypertrophy.

• **Direct vasodilators,** such as sodium nitroprusside, intravenous nitrates, hydralazine, diazoxide, and minoxidil, cause peripheral vasodilation directly. This usually results in reflex tachycardia. Prolonged intravenous sodium nitroprusside administration causes toxic thiocyanate concentrations and, after 48 h, levels should be monitored.

• **Centrally acting drugs,** such as clonidine, methyldopa, and guanethidine, are seldom used as a result of multiple side effects.

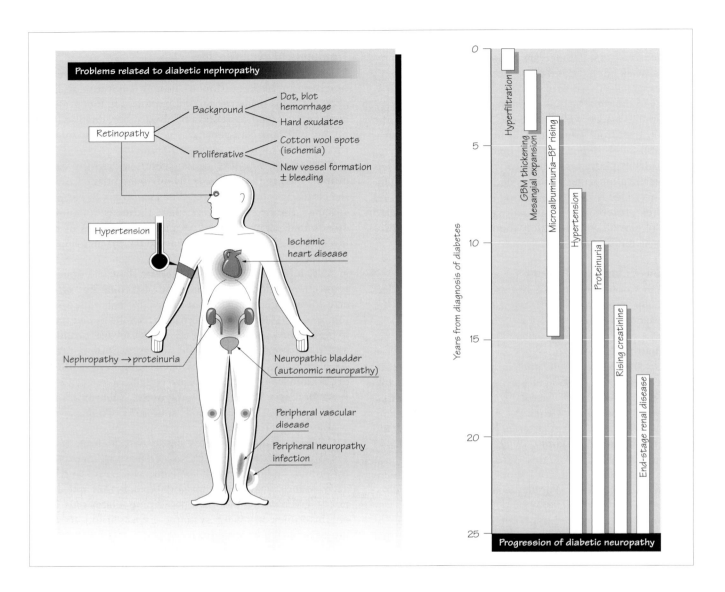

Between 25% and 50% of all patients with diabetes develop nephropathy. Diabetes is the most common single cause of end-stage renal disease and accounts for 30–40% of all cases.

Clinical progression of diabetic nephropathy

A minority of patients, especially those with poor glycemic control, already have enlarged kidneys with an increased glomerular filtration rate (GFR) at the time that their diabetes is diagnosed. This hyperfiltration may result from intraglomerular hypertension caused by preferential efferent arteriolar constriction. The next renal abnormality to develop is microalbuminuria (20–200 µg/min), which is

below the threshold of conventional dipsticks. Microalbuminuria is a strong predictor of subsequent nephropathy and is associated with mild hypertension and mild insulin resistance. After a period of microalbuminuria, patients may progress to overt nephropathy, with hypertension, dipstick proteinuria (>0.5 g/24 h) and a linear decline in GFR. Severe proteinuria can cause the nephrotic syndrome. Most patients with nephropathy also have retinopathy and hyperlipidemia. If retinopathy is present, a renal biopsy is not usually necessary but, if it is absent, other causes of renal disease, especially renal artery stenosis, should be excluded.

Microvascular changes in diabetic kidneys are typical of

diabetic changes occurring elsewhere, such as in the retina. The vessel walls become thickened with glycosylated matrix, and in some cases vessel occlusion develops. These changes impair oxygen diffusion out of the vessel, causing tissue ischemia. In the retina this leads to new vessel formation. In patients with non-insulin-dependent diabetes mellitus (NIDDM), nephropathy is less common in those of European descent than in those of African or Asian descent. It takes about 15–20 years from the onset of proteinuria to develop end-stage renal disease, but many patients with NIDDM die before this as a result of cardiovascular disease.

Factors promoting nephropathy in people with diabetes

The Diabetes Control and Complications Trial showed that good glycemic control slows the rate at which proteinuria develops and progresses. Hyperglycemia causes protein glycosylation which promotes protein cross-linking. Cross-linking could either interfere with collagen molecules of the glomerular basement membrane or trigger mesangial cells to secrete the excess extracellular matrix that is present. Increased intraglomerular pressure causes early hyperfiltration and may also damage the endothelium and glomerular filtration barrier. Growth-promoting hormones, such as growth hormone, insulin-like growth factor, and platelet-derived growth factors, may promote the early renal hypertrophy and trigger the accompanying renal hemodynamic changes. There is a familial tendency to nephropathy in both IDDM and NIDDM. Candidate genes include the red cell sodium/lithium co-transporter, the red cell sodium/hydrogen counter-transporter, and the angiotensin-converting enzyme (ACE).

Histologic changes

The glomerular basement membrane is thickened with deposition of albumin and other plasma proteins within it. There is mesangial expansion causing loss of filtration surface. Afferent and efferent arterioles undergo hyalinosis as a result of the deposition of lipid and glycoprotein material in the arterial wall. Nodular exudative lesions and diffuse glomerulosclerosis represent long-standing nephropathy.

Treatment

Pre-end-stage renal disease

Patients with diabetes should be monitored for microalbuminuria at least once a year. If microalbuminuria is detected, ACE inhibitors have been shown to reduce proteinuria and reduce the probability of progression to end-stage renal disease. Strict blood pressure control can also reduce proteinuria and progression to end-stage renal disease. Good glycemic control reduces the probability of microvascular complications such as nephropathy in IDDM. If renal impairment develops in NIDDM, only short-acting hypoglycemic drugs metabolized by the liver, such as gliclazide and tolbutamide, should be used. Other drugs may accumulate and biguanides can cause lactic acidosis.

End-stage renal disease

People with diabetes who have end-stage renal disease have a higher mortality than patients who do not have diabetes but have end-stage renal disease, irrespective of the mode of renal replacement therapy. The main causes of death are cardiovascular disease and infection. Renal transplantation offers the best prognosis and quality of life. Some units perform routine coronary angiography and revascularization before renal transplantation, because of the high incidence of coronary artery disease. Diabetic foot problems, caused by a combination of peripheral vascular disease, peripheral neuropathy, and infection, are especially common after transplantation and can result in the need to amputate. Combined kidney and pancreas transplantations are increasingly performed in patients who have diabetic nephropathy. Rejection rates are higher than for kidneys alone and more immunosuppression is required, but the quality of life is usually much improved if the transplantation is successful.

The half-life of insulin is increased with severe renal impairment. Insulin requirements fall and there is an increased risk of hypoglycemia. Altered red cell survival on hemodialysis or peritoneal dialysis makes glycated hemoglobin measurements unreliable and regular home monitoring of glucose is preferable. It is possible to put insulin into peritoneal dialysis bags to provide glycemic control, avoiding subcutaneous injection of insulin. Retinopathy and blindness can affect the patient's ability to perform peritoneal dialysis.

Other renal problems related to diabetes

Diabetes can contribute to papillary ischemia, especially if there is also infection or abuse of analgesics. The result is papillary necrosis (see Chapter 32) with sloughing of the papilla and often hematuria and pyuria. Urinary tract infection is more common in people with diabetes and a contributory factor can be incomplete voiding of urine, resulting from autonomic neuropathy.

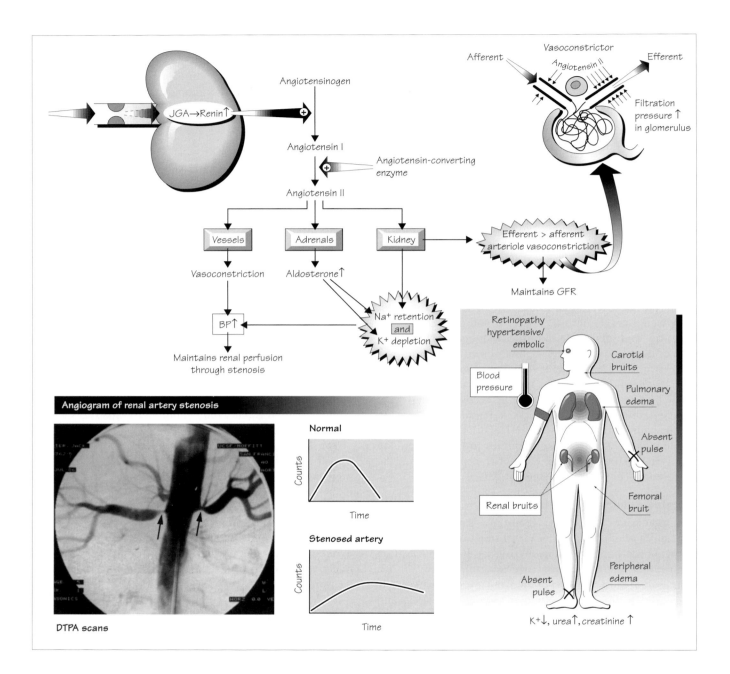

Angiotensinogen

JGA→Renin↑

Angiotensin I

Angiotensin-converting enzyme

Angiotensin II

Vessels | Adrenals | Kidney

Vasoconstriction

Aldosterone↑

Na+ retention and K+ depletion

BP↑

Maintains renal perfusion through stenosis

Efferent > afferent arteriole vasoconstriction

Maintains GFR

Afferent | Vasoconstrictor Angiotensin II | Efferent

Filtration pressure ↑ in glomerulus

Angiogram of renal artery stenosis

DTPA scans

Normal

Counts

Time

Stenosed artery

Counts

Time

Retinopathy hypertensive/ embolic

Blood pressure

Carotid bruits

Pulmonary edema

Absent pulse

Renal bruits

Femoral bruit

Absent pulse

Peripheral edema

K+↓, urea↑, creatinine ↑

Renal artery stenosis reduces the renal blood flow and glomerular filtration, causing renal ischemia, hypertension, and sodium and water retention. The main causes are atherosclerosis in older patients and fibromuscular dysplasia in young patients. Renal artery stenosis accounts for 1–5% of all hypertension. Atherosclerotic disease is often bilateral and usually progresses, sometimes to complete occlusion. Fibromuscular dysplasia does not usually cause occlusion.

Renal artery stenosis — pathophysiology
Hypertension
Decreased renal perfusion stimulates the juxtaglomerular apparatus to release renin, which enhances angiotensin II production. Angiotensin II causes hypertension by systemic vasoconstriction and by stimulating aldosterone release, which promotes salt and water retention.

Renal impairment

Angiotensin II vasoconstricts the efferent arterioles more than the afferent arterioles. This reduces renal blood flow, but maintains glomerular filtration, so the filtration fraction is increased. Inhibition of angiotensin II (with angiotensin II antagonists or angiotensin-converting enzyme or ACE inhibitors) removes the efferent arteriolar constriction causing a fall in the glomerular filtration rate (GFR). Microembolization from an atheromatous plaque can contribute to renal damage. If only one kidney has a stenosed artery, plasma creatinine may be normal because of compensatory hyperfiltration by the other kidney.

Edema

Bilateral renal artery disease causes enhanced proximal tubular sodium reabsorption. Contributory factors include a fall in renal blood flow, stimulation of the proximal tubule Na^+/H^+ exchanger by angiotensin II, and stimulation of distal tubular sodium reabsorption by aldosterone. Aldosterone also promotes potassium secretion which can cause hypokalemia. Mild proteinuria can occur, possibly because angiotensin II increases glomerular pore size. In unilateral renal artery stenosis, salt and water balance are normalized by the other kidney.

Etiology of renal artery stenosis

Atherosclerotic disease usually affects the proximal renal artery and accounts for most cases. There is often vascular disease elsewhere and the usual risk factors for atherosclerosis—smoking, diabetes mellitus, hypertension, a family history, and hyperlipidemia. **Fibromuscular dysplasia** occurs in younger patients, especially women. It can occur as multiple bands separated by dilated segments, appearing like a string of beads on an angiogram. **Rare causes** of renal artery stenosis include Takayasu's inflammatory arteritis, neurofibromatosis, pressure from renal artery aneurysms, and extrinsic pressure.

History and examination

There may be a history of risk factors for atherosclerosis or symptoms of vascular disease elsewhere. *A rapid deterioration in renal function caused by an ACE inhibitor is highly suggestive.* There is often hypertension and signs of vascular disease elsewhere, such as absent pulses, aneurysms, or arterial bruits. Bruits caused by turbulent flow through a stenosed renal artery may be heard over the kidneys. Hypertensive retinopathy may be present and there may be pulmonary or peripheral edema.

Investigation

The diagnosis is suggested by hypokalemia, elevated urea and creatinine, and different sized kidneys on ultrasonography. With unilateral disease, ischemic damage reduces the size of the affected kidney. The definitive investigation is angiography through an arterial catheter introduced at the groin or in the arm. Non-invasive imaging techniques such as magnetic resonance angiography and Doppler ultrasonography are improving. **^{99m}Tc-labeled DTPA** (technetium-99m-labeled diethylenetriaminepenta-acetic acid) is freely filtered at the glomerulus and neither secreted nor reabsorbed. After injection, a gamma camera produces a curve showing isotope accumulation in each kidney. In renal artery stenosis, angiotensin II increases proximal tubular sodium and therefore water reabsorption. This reduces urine flow which delays the peak and slows the downward phase. Furosemide given during the scan increases the specificity for enhanced proximal reabsorption, by inhibiting excess distal salt reabsorption. Administration of an ACE inhibitor during the renogram removes the effect of angiotensin II (which also maintains the GFR) and makes the test more sensitive.

Treatment

ACE inhibitors can reduce the GFR and are usually avoided. A unilateral fall may be undetected by serum creatinine measurement. Aspirin may prevent thrombus formation at the stenosis. Percutaneous transluminal balloon angioplasty, sometimes with the insertion of an expandable stent, is standard therapy. The success rate is higher for fibromuscular dysplasia than for atherosclerotic disease. The response of hypertension to relief of the stenosis is variable. Very rarely, uncontrollable hypertension requires renal embolization or nephrectomy to remove the source of renin.

Cholesterol emboli

Detached fragments of atheroma in the aorta or renal arteries can embolize to the kidneys, especially after arterial surgery or angiographic instrumentation. Microemboli of cholesterol crystals and debris provoke an inflammation and fibrosis. Showers of these crystals can also cause *livedo reticularis* in the legs or microembolic lesions in the retina.

Renal vein thrombosis

Thrombus in the renal veins or their tributaries reduces the renal blood flow and impairs renal function. This may be clinically silent, although flank pain, loin tenderness, and macroscopic hematuria can occur. Diagnosis is made by renal venography, but may be evident using Doppler flow studies or computed tomography or magnetic resonance imaging. Any prothrombotic state can cause renal vein thrombosis. In nephrotic syndrome, renal vein thrombosis impairs renal function, increases proteinuria, and almost always causes microscopic hematuria. Renal vein thrombosis can extend and occlude the inferior vena cava or cause pulmonary emboli.

38 Polycystic kidney disease

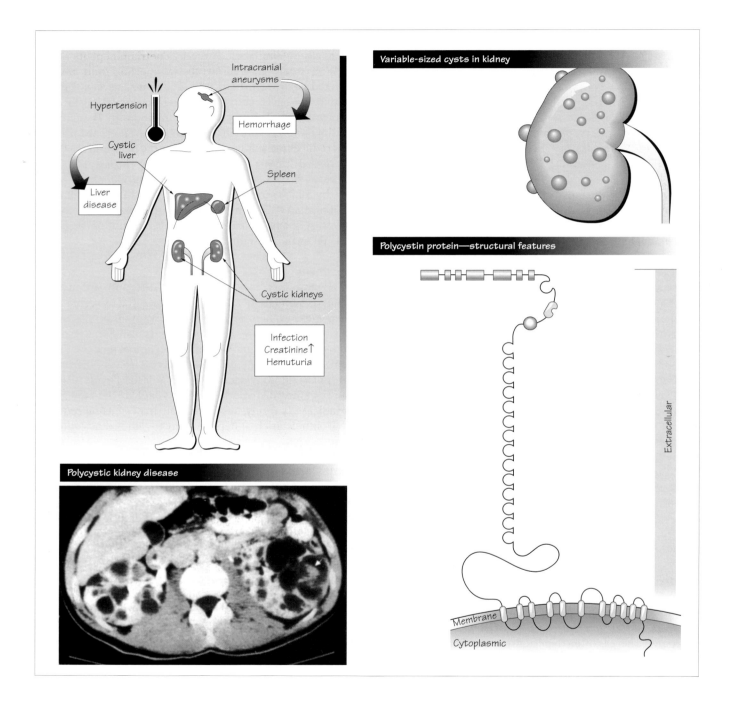

Intracranial aneurysms
Hypertension
Hemorrhage
Cystic liver
Liver disease
Spleen
Cystic kidneys
Infection
Creatinine↑
Hemuturia

Polycystic kidney disease

Variable-sized cysts in kidney

Polycystin protein—structural features

Extracellular

Membrane
Cytoplasmic

Autosomal dominant polycystic kidney disease (ADPKD) is the most common inherited kidney disorder. The prevalence is around 1 in 1000 and it is more common in white than in black populations. It accounts for 4–10% of patients with kidney failure requiring dialysis or transplantation. The disease results from mutations in one of three separate loci. Candidate genes for two of these loci have been identified and are known as the *PKD1* and *PKD2* genes. *PKD2*-related disease seems to progress more slowly than *PKD1*-related disease.

The key clinical features are multiple cysts in the kidneys, but there may also be cysts in the liver, spleen, and pancreas.

Intracranial aneurysms and cardiac valve abnormalities can also occur. The cysts arise *in utero* and slowly destroy the surrounding normal tissue as they grow throughout adult life. Although the disease can be asymptomatic, symptoms can result from the presence of the cysts themselves or the effect of the disease on renal function. The cysts can cause pain directly or pain can arise from bleeding into the cysts, infection, or renal stones. High blood pressure is common and may contribute to the reduced life expectancy.

Clinical disease
Renal abnormalities
There are multiple cysts in both kidneys, which can be visualized by ultrasonography, computed tomography (CT), or magnetic resonance imaging (MRI). Cysts vary in size from microscopic to several centimeters in diameter. The cysts are fluid filled and prone to secondary complications. Distended cysts can cause chronic pain. Bleeding into a cyst can result in acute pain and hematuria. Cysts can become infected and sometimes develop into abscesses.

Renal stone formation is common and may result from urinary stasis which occurs as a consequence of the cysts. High blood pressure is common and can occur before renal function deteriorates. The reason for this hypertension is not clear. Progressive renal failure is common but does not occur in all patients and the rate of deterioration varies, even within families. By the age of 50, about 50% of affected individuals have renal failure.

Extrarenal manifestations
Around 50% of patients have cysts in the liver. Although liver function is usually normal, large cysts can cause liver damage and abdominal problems. Cysts in the spleen, pancreas, and other organs are usually asymptomatic. The incidence of intracranial aneurysms is increased in ADPKD and these can rupture, resulting in subarachnoid hemorrhage. A number of patients have cardiac valvular incompetence, especially of the mitral and tricuspid valves. Anemia is less common in patients with renal failure caused by ADPKD than it is in other patients with renal failure, because there is sustained erythropoietin production by the kidneys, possibly from the cysts.

Diagnosis
Patients can present with hematuria or pain in the loin or abdomen. More commonly, the diagnosis is made during the investigation of abnormal renal function, hypertension, urinary infection, or stones. There is generally a family history and physical examination may reveal large palpable kidneys (and sometimes liver and spleen) and hypertension. Prenatal diagnosis is now possible for some affected families.

Treatment
There is no specific treatment. High blood pressure and infection should be treated conventionally. If renal failure develops, dialysis or transplantation is required.

Juvenile disease
Although classic ADPKD can manifest itself in children, children can also present with the much rarer autosomal recessive polycystic kidney disease.

Molecular pathology
PKD1
The *PKD1* gene is on the short arm of chromosome 16 and mutations in this gene account for about 90% of cases of ADPKD. The gene is large, with 46 exons, and it encodes polycystin, a protein consisting of 4304 amino acids. Polycystin contains a number of recognizable motifs including a C-type lectin carbohydrate recognition domain, an LDL-A (low-density lipoprotein A-like) domain, various immunoglobulin-like domains, and 11 probable transmembrane domains. The protein could play a multifunctional role in cell–cell or cell–matrix adhesion and recognition. It could also be an ion channel regulator.

Cysts
Cysts arise from any segment of the nephron or collecting duct. They may arise because tubular epithelial cells lose their normal polarization. Certainly, the Na^+/K^+ ATPase that is normally restricted to the basolateral surface of tubular epithelial cells is present on the apical surface of abnormal cystic epithelia. Analysis of cells isolated from individual cysts has suggested that most cysts are clonally derived, implying derivation from a single cell. As the disease is dominant, affected individuals are heterozygotes, but many cysts are no longer heterozygous, and have lost their normal allele. It may be that both germline and somatic mutations are required for cyst formation and growth.

PKD2
The *PKD2* gene is on the long arm of chromosome 4 and accounts for around 10% of patients with ADPKD. The gene encodes a protein of 968 amino acids with a molecular mass of 110 kDa, which has homology with a voltage-gated calcium channel. There are probably six membrane-spanning regions. Unlike polycystin, the protein does not appear to be suitable for cell–cell or cell–matrix interactions. However, the PKD2 protein has extensive homology with polycystin and with a family of voltage-gated calcium and sodium channels.

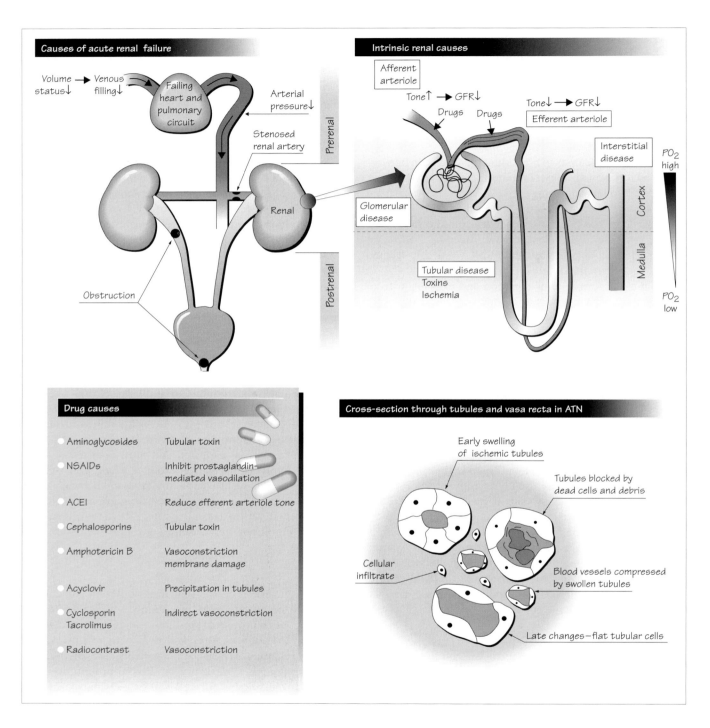

Causes of acute renal failure

Volume status↓ → Venous filling↓ → Failing heart and pulmonary circuit

Arterial pressure↓

Stenosed renal artery

Renal

Prerenal

Postrenal

Obstruction

Intrinsic renal causes

Afferent arteriole

Tone↑ → GFR↓

Drugs

Drugs

Tone↓ → GFR↓

Efferent arteriole

Interstitial disease

Glomerular disease

Tubular disease
Toxins
Ischemia

Cortex

Medulla

PO₂ high

PO₂ low

Drug causes

Aminoglycosides	Tubular toxin
NSAIDs	Inhibit prostaglandin-mediated vasodilation
ACEI	Reduce efferent arteriole tone
Cephalosporins	Tubular toxin
Amphotericin B	Vasoconstriction membrane damage
Acyclovir	Precipitation in tubules
Cyclosporin Tacrolimus	Indirect vasoconstriction
Radiocontrast	Vasoconstriction

Cross-section through tubules and vasa recta in ATN

Early swelling of ischemic tubules

Tubules blocked by dead cells and debris

Cellular infiltrate

Blood vessels compressed by swollen tubules

Late changes—flat tubular cells

Acute renal failure arises when there is an acute fall in glomerular filtration rate (GFR) and substances that are usually excreted by the kidneys accumulate in the blood. Acute renal failure can be caused by inadequate renal perfusion (prerenal), intrinsic renal disease (renal), and urinary tract obstruction (postrenal). Prerenal conditions account for 50–65% of cases, postrenal for 15%, and renal for the remaining 20–35%. In developing countries, obstetric complications and infections such as malaria are important causes. The overall mortality rate is around 30–70%, depending on age and the presence of other organ failure or disease. Of survivors, 60% regain normal renal function, but 15–30% have renal impairment and around 5–10% develop end-stage renal disease.

Prerenal disease

Inadequate cardiac function, circulatory volume depletion, and obstruction of the arterial supply to the kidneys can all impair renal perfusion. The resulting renal ischemia can cause acute tubular necrosis (ATN).

Postrenal disease

Obstruction to urine flow causes back-pressure which inhibits filtration. The subsequent swelling compresses blood vessels causing ischemia. Acute renal failure arises only if both kidneys are obstructed or if there is only one kidney and that kidney is obstructed. The cause of the obstruction can be within the urinary tract (such as a stone), within the wall of the tract (such as a tumor or stricture), or outside the wall (such as compression by a mass or fibrotic process).

Intrinsic renal disease

Intrinsic renal causes of acute renal failure are glomerular disease, tubulointerstitial disease, and drugs or toxins. The main *glomerular* causes of acute renal failure are acute or rapidly progressive glomerulonephritis, Goodpasture's syndrome, vasculitis, and proliferative glomerulonephritis associated with a multisystem disease or infection.

Tubular toxins

Tubular injury can result from ischemia, or from toxic effects of exogenous compounds such as drugs, heavy metals, and contrast media or endogenous compounds such as hemoglobin or myoglobin. Exercise, trauma, or other causes of muscle damage cause rhabdomyolysis with myoglobin release. Hemolysis destroys red cells, releasing hemoglobin. Hemolytic uremic syndrome consists of hemolysis and acute renal failure and can follow infection with *Escherichia coli* serotype 0157:H7. Both hemoglobin and myoglobin are filtered in the glomerulus and are toxic to tubular cells. Acute hypercalcemia can cause acute renal failure by renal vasoconstriction, but also by calcium phosphate precipitation in the tubules. In myeloma, light chain precipitation in the tubules can cause acute renal failure.

Drugs

Any drug can cause an allergic tubulointerstitial nephritis, especially non-steroidal anti-inflammatory drugs (NSAIDs), diuretics, and antibiotics (see Chapter 32). Some drugs cause renal failure through other mechanisms (see figure).

NSAIDs. Normally there is a tonic prostaglandin-induced vasodilation of renal arterioles. NSAIDs inhibit prostaglandin synthesis. This leads to vasoconstriction which reduces renal blood flow. If there is volume depletion, the vasoconstrictive drive may be very strong, causing a serious fall in GFR. Risk factors for NSAID-induced renal failure are volume depletion, diuretic use, pre-existing renal impairment, and an edema state (congestive heart failure, liver cirrhosis, or nephrotic syndrome). **Aminoglycoside antibiotics** are tubular toxins which cause acute tubular necrosis. In renal artery stenosis (see Chapter 37 renal artery stenosis), angiotensin II causes efferent arteriolar constriction to maintain the GFR. An **angiotensin-converting enzyme inhibitor** can block this constriction, causing a large fall in the GFR.

Pathophysiology of acute tubular necrosis

Most acute renal failure results from ATN. This usually arises when there is renal hypoperfusion, with renal ischaemia, in combination with other factors such as sepsis or circulating tubular toxins or nephrotoxic drugs. ATN is associated with tubular cell death and shedding into the tubular lumen, resulting in tubular blockage (see Chapter 32). This raises the tubular pressure which eventually stops further glomerular filtration. Swollen tubules also compress the nearby vasa recta, which further reduces perfusion.

Vascular effects of ischemia

Various factors can exacerbate ischemia, including disordered regulation of vascular tone after an initial ischemic insult. Ischemic renal endothelium releases the vasoconstrictor endothelin. As well as increased levels of vasoconstrictors, including angiotensin II, catecholamines, and arachidonic acid metabolites, there may be low levels of locally acting vasodilators such as prostacyclin (PGI_2) and nitric oxide (NO). Initially, tubular damage reduces sodium reabsorption. This increases tubular sodium concentrations at the macula densa, stimulating renin secretion and vasoconstriction via angiotensin II (see Chapter 13).

Cellular mechanisms of tubular damage

A number of mechanisms are implicated in the process of tubular injury. Ischemia causes production of *oxygen free radicals*. These damage cellular and mitochondrial membrane lipids and can lead to cell death. Ischemia depletes ATP and so *inhibits energy-dependent calcium efflux* from cells. Elevated intracellular calcium levels interfere with metabolic processes. Ischemic cells can *lose their actin cytoskeletal integrity* and detach from the basement membrane. Ischemic cells can also lose their membrane polarity, allowing channels to move around the membrane which disrupts tubular transport function. Apoptosis and necrosis of tubular cells are common.

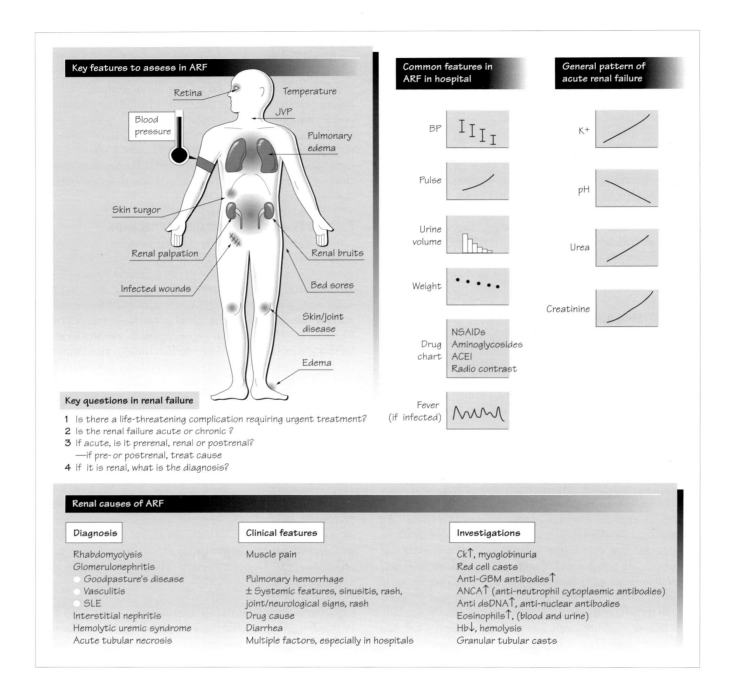

Key features to assess in ARF

- Retina
- Temperature
- JVP
- Blood pressure
- Pulmonary edema
- Skin turgor
- Renal palpation
- Renal bruits
- Infected wounds
- Bed sores
- Skin/joint disease
- Edema

Key questions in renal failure

1 Is there a life-threatening complication requiring urgent treatment?
2 Is the renal failure acute or chronic ?
3 If acute, is it prerenal, renal or postrenal?
— if pre- or postrenal, treat cause
4 If it is renal, what is the diagnosis?

Common features in ARF in hospital

- BP
- Pulse
- Urine volume
- Weight
- Drug chart: NSAIDs, Aminoglycosides, ACEI, Radio contrast
- Fever (if infected)

General pattern of acute renal failure

- K+
- pH
- Urea
- Creatinine

Renal causes of ARF

Diagnosis	Clinical features	Investigations
Rhabdomyolysis	Muscle pain	Ck↑, myoglobinuria
Glomerulonephritis		Red cell casts
● Goodpasture's disease	Pulmonary hemorrhage	Anti-GBM antibodies↑
● Vasculitis	± Systemic features, sinusitis, rash,	ANCA↑ (anti-neutrophil cytoplasmic antibodies)
● SLE	joint/neurological signs, rash	Anti dsDNA↑, anti-nuclear antibodies
Interstitial nephritis	Drug cause	Eosinophils↑, (blood and urine)
Hemolytic uremic syndrome	Diarrhea	Hb↓, hemolysis
Acute tubular necrosis	Multiple factors, especially in hospitals	Granular tubular casts

Most acute renal failure arises in hospital from fluid depletion, sepsis or drug toxicity, especially after surgery, trauma, or burns. There is usually a fall in urine output and a rise in serum urea and creatinine. A urine output of less than 400 mL/day is termed oliguria.

History

A history may indicate pre-existing renal impairment, hypertension, or diabetes which all predispose to renal ischemia. Frank hematuria followed by oliguria suggests glomerulonephritis; hemoptysis suggests Goodpasture's syndrome; a recent throat or skin infection suggests post-infectious glomerulonephritis. In men, urinary frequency, nocturia, and a poor stream with hesitancy and dribbling suggest postrenal obstruction resulting from prostate disease. Muscle pain and swelling after exercise suggest rhabdomyolysis. Recent gastroenteritis can indicate *Escherichia coli*-associated hemolytic uremic syndrome. The **past medical history** may reveal an underlying multisystem disease associated with glomerulonephritis, vascular disease (associated with renal artery stenosis), malignancy (associated with hypercalcemia), or chronic infection such as osteomyelitis or abnormal heart valves that are vulnerable to endocarditis. The **drug history** should include possible self-poisoning and analgesic use.

Examination

Assess the fluid volume status. Look for signs of a multisystem disease, of cholesterol emboli, and of intravenous drug use. Muscle swelling or tenderness suggests rhabdomyolysis. The eyes may have hypertensive, diabetic, or other diagnostic changes. Examine all bed sores, and surgical and traumatic wounds for sepsis. Pulse, blood pressure (lying and standing if necessary), jugular venous pressure, and a cardiac examination may indicate volume depletion, cardiac lesions, or a pericarditis. Examine the chest for pulmonary edema and evidence of infection or bleeding. Upper airway disease or sinusitis suggests Wegener's disease. Polycystic kidneys may be palpable and a large palpable bladder suggests obstruction. Rectal examination may demonstrate prostate or pelvic disease.

Investigations

Blood biochemistry. Hyperkalemia and severe acidosis can cause cardiac arrest. In rhabdomyolysis, plasma creatine kinase levels are high because it is released from muscle.

Hematology. Anemia can result from blood loss, suppressed erythropoiesis, low erythropoietin levels, or hemolysis. A high eosinophil count suggests acute interstitial nephritis. Hemolytic uremic syndrome causes hemolysis with anemia, damaged red blood cells, and a low platelet count.

Urine. Urine microscopy and culture should be performed. Heavy proteinuria suggests glomerulonephritis or myeloma. Hematuria indicates renal or postrenal disease, but can be caused by urinary catheterization. Myoglobin in the urine suggests rhabdomyolysis, and hemoglobin suggests hemolysis. Granular tubular casts may occur in acute tubular necrosis. Red cell casts are diagnostic of glomerular disease. Eosinophils in the urine suggest interstitial nephritis.

Radiology. Ultrasonography is mandatory to exclude obstruction and to determine the size of the kidneys. Small kidneys indicate chronic renal failure. Angiography or ultrasonographic Doppler studies or radio-isotopic methods can evaluate renal perfusion.

Immunology. Complement levels are low in systemic lupus erythematosus and post-infectious glomerulonephritis. Anti-glomerular basement membrane antibody suggests Goodpasture's syndrome and antineutrophil cytoplasmic antibodies (ANCAs) suggest vasculitis. Antinuclear antibodies or antibodies to double-stranded DNA suggest systemic lupus erythematosus.

Microbiology and histology. Cultures should be taken to exclude sepsis and, if the etiology of renal disease is unclear, a renal biopsy should be performed.

Management

Prerenal or postrenal causes must be corrected urgently. Intrinsic renal disease is treated according to its type. Regardless of the etiology, certain basic measures are routine.

Electrolytes. Plasma electrolytes should be measured daily. Potassium intake should be restricted and diuretics or renal replacement therapy used to prevent hyperkalemia.

Acid. Acid inhibits metabolic processes. Severe acidosis with inadequate renal function must be treated with renal replacement therapy.

Volume. Regularly assess the body volume. When necessary, measure the central venous pressure with an internal jugular or subclavian venous catheter. Monitor the fluid intake and output. Urinary catheterization provides accurate urine volumes, but is an infection risk. Daily insensible losses vary with a minimum of 500 mL and around 500 mL extra per °C of fever. Daily weighing of patients can guide volume replacement. Volume replacement should match known and insensible losses.

Pulmonary edema. The patient should be sat up and given oxygen. Diuretics are given if there is any renal function. If not, renal replacement therapy must be instituted urgently. In the meantime, nitrates and opiates provide vasodilation. If necessary venesect 200–500 mL blood and ventilate the patient with positive end-expiratory pressures.

General measures

Correct any hypoxia with oxygen and, if necessary, ventilation. Cardiac output should be maintained with inotropes. Hemoglobin should be kept above 10 g/dL to maintain tissue oxygenation. Patients are often hypercatabolic and must be fed nasogastrically or parenterally if they cannot eat. Hypertension should be controlled by adjusting fluid balance and antihypertensives if necessary.

Renal replacement therapy

Absolute indications for renal replacement therapy include hyperkalemia, acidosis, pulmonary edema, and severe uremic complications. Hemodialysis is poorly tolerated by hemodynamically unstable patients. Continuous hemofiltration which is slower is better tolerated.

41

Chronic renal failure and renal bone disease

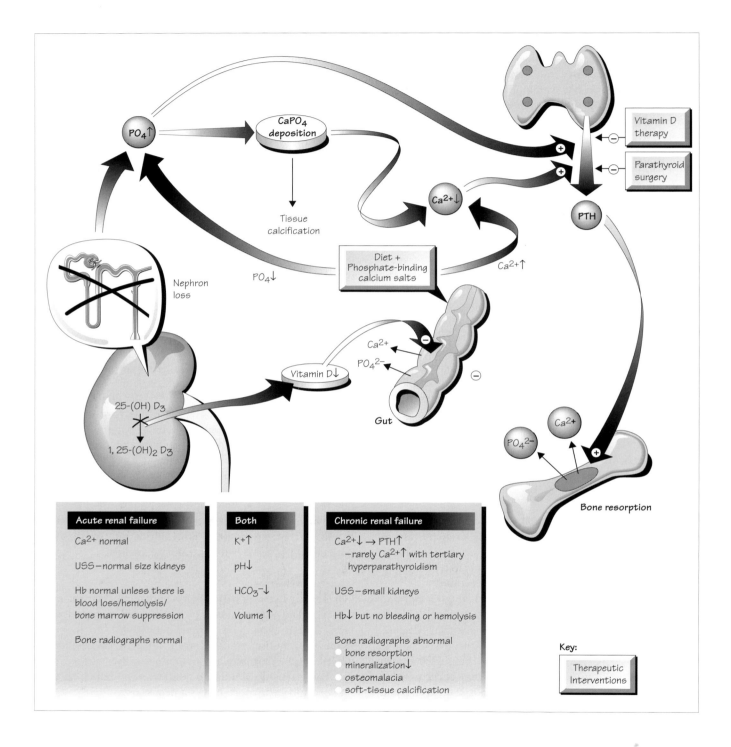

Any disease process causing progressive nephron loss can cause chronic renal failure. As the number of functioning nephrons declines, the surviving nephrons compensate by increasing filtration and solute reabsorption. Unfortu- nately, this damages the remaining nephrons and acceler- ates nephron loss. *End-stage renal disease* occurs when patients require renal replacement therapy with dialysis or transplantation.

Complications of chronic renal failure are caused by the accumulation of substances that are normally excreted by the kidney, and by inadequate production of vitamin D and erythropoietin by the kidney. The *uremic syndrome* refers to the complications of chronic renal failure such as anemia, confusion, coma, asterixis, seizures, pericardial effusion, itch, and bone disease. Renal replacement therapy improves these problems, but patients with end-stage renal disease have a higher morbidity and mortality than the rest of the population.

Distinction between acute and chronic renal failure

Both acute and chronic renal failure raise plasma potassium, urea, and creatinine, and cause metabolic acidosis. In chronic renal failure there is usually evidence of chronic complications, including anemia caused by inadequate erythropoietin, and bone disease, typically with a low calcium, a raised phosphate, and a high parathyroid hormone (PTH) level. Plasma calcium is characteristically low in chronic renal failure, unless tertiary hyperparathyroidism is present (see Chapter 24). The key finding in chronic renal failure is small kidneys on ultrasonography. The reduction in size is caused by atrophy and fibrosis.

Acute problems in chronic renal failure

Acute problems can occur in both acute and chronic renal failure. Emergency treatment with dialysis or hemofiltration may be needed for life-threatening hyperkalemia, severe acidosis, pulmonary edema, and uremic symptoms. Sudden deterioration in patients with renal impairment who are not yet on dialysis can be triggered by severe hypertension, urinary tract infection, or nephrotoxic drugs. Non-steroidal anti-inflammatory drugs or angiotensin-converting enzyme inhibitors can cause renal deterioration by adversely affecting glomerular blood flow.

Renal bone disease and calcium and phosphate metabolism

Renal bone disease can cause bone pain, especially in the lower back, hips, and legs, and is often associated with proximal myopathy and soft tissue calcification. Bone alkaline phosphatase is usually elevated. Two types of renal bone disease can be distinguished by bone biopsy. Most renal bone disease is conventional or **high-turnover bone disease** in which there is excess PTH. The PTH stimulates bone resorption and the new bone that replaces it has disordered collagen. Radiographs may show subperiosteal resorption in the phalanges, erosion of the phalangeal tufts, and erosion of the clavicle heads. In **low-turnover bone disease**, PTH levels are low. Bone turnover is low and there is osteomalacia with poorly mineralized bone. This bone disease arises if calcium intake and plasma calcium levels are high enough to suppress PTH secretion below the level required for healthy bone turnover. Vitamin D levels may

also be low. Radiographs may show multiple fractures or pseudofractures (radiolucent cortical zones perpendicular to the bone surface).

Causes of high-turnover renal bone disease

The main causes of renal bone disease are renal phosphate retention and inadequate renal vitamin D production. Vitamin D deficiency reduces calcium and phosphate absorption but, when renal phosphate retention also occurs, the net result is a rise in phosphate and a fall in calcium. The rise in phosphate further lowers the calcium by causing calcium phosphate deposition in tissues. The hypocalcemia stimulates a rise in PTH, causing secondary hyperparathyroidism (see Chapter 24). Eventually, PTH secretion can become autonomous and fail to fall even if calcium rises as a result of bone mobilization. This is termed tertiary hyperparathyroidism. Other factors can exacerbate renal bone disease. A high phosphate level directly stimulates PTH secretion and directly inhibits renal vitamin D production. Normally, vitamin D binds to receptors on parathyroid cells and inhibits PTH secretion, so vitamin D deficiency causes excess PTH secretion. Acidosis stimulates bone resorption.

Treatment of high-turnover renal bone disease

Dialysis removes some phosphate from the plasma. However, for proper phosphate control, dietary phosphate intake should be reduced and phosphate-binding calcium salts taken with food. These salts bind dietary phosphate, blocking its absorption in the gut. Vitamin D given as 1,25-dihydroxy-vitamin D_3 [1,25-$(OH)_2$-D_3 or calcitriol] or 1-hydroxy-vitamin D_3 [1-(OH)-D_3 or alfacalcidol] inhibits PTH secretion and bone turnover, and raises plasma calcium by increasing dietary calcium absorption. It may also help bone pain and proximal myopathy. Treatment should reduce PTH levels sufficiently to prevent high-turnover bone disease without causing adynamic low-turnover bone disease. If PTH does not fall when calcium levels rise and vitamin D is administered, surgery to remove most or all of the parathyroid glands is indicated. Bone disease may also improve with rigorous correction of acidosis by dialysis and sometimes administration of calcium carbonate or sodium bicarbonate between dialyses.

Table 41.1 Most common causes requiring renal replacement therapy.

Cause	%
Diabetes mellitus	40
Hypertension	25
Glomerulonephritis	15
Polycystic kidney disease	4
Urologic	6
Unknown and miscellaneous	10

42

Chronic renal failure: clinical complications and their management

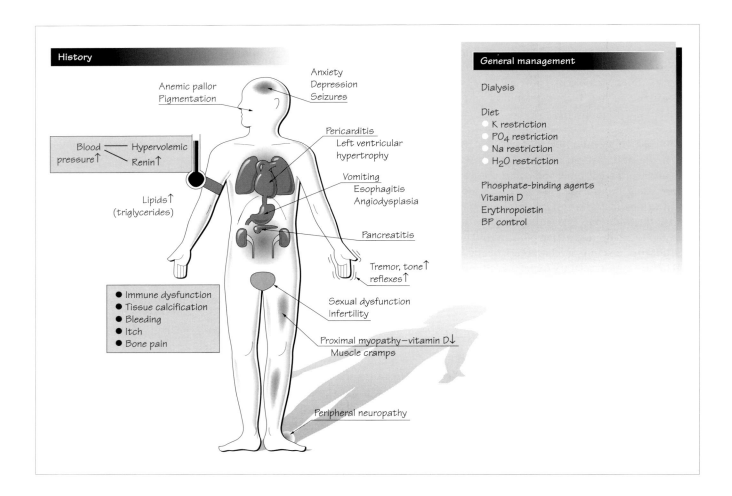

History

Anemic pallor
Pigmentation

Anxiety
Depression
Seizures

Blood pressure↑ — Hypervolemic
Renin↑

Pericarditis
Left ventricular hypertrophy

Lipids↑
(triglycerides)

Vomiting
Esophagitis
Angiodysplasia

Pancreatitis

Tremor, tone↑
reflexes↑

● Immune dysfunction
● Tissue calcification
● Bleeding
● Itch
● Bone pain

Sexual dysfunction
Infertility

Proximal myopathy—vitamin D↓
Muscle cramps

Peripheral neuropathy

General management

Dialysis

Diet
○ K restriction
○ PO_4 restriction
○ Na restriction
○ H_2O restriction

Phosphate-binding agents
Vitamin D
Erythropoietin
BP control

Many complications arise as renal function declines. Renal bone disease is considered in Chapter 41.

Hematologic complications

Anemia in chronic renal disease is caused by inadequate erythropoietin production by the kidney (see Chapter 12) and is treated by giving erythropoietin subcutaneously or intravenously. This works only if iron, folate, and vitamin B_{12} levels are adequate and the patient is otherwise well.

Although laboratory clotting times are normal, platelet function is impaired and the **bleeding time** (the time for bleeding from a cut to stop) is increased. The bleeding time can be improved by efficient dialysis, correction of anemia with erythropoietin, and administration of conjugated estrogens. Synthetic vasopressin (desmopressin or DDAVP) increases factor VIII (von Willebrand's factor) levels and transiently reduces the bleeding time.

Vascular disease and hypertension

Vascular disease is the major cause of death in chronic renal failure. In patients who do not have diabetes, hypertension is probably the most important risk factor. Most hypertension in chronic renal disease results from the hypervolemia caused by sodium and water retention. This is not usually severe enough to cause edema, but there may be a triple cardiac rhythm. Such hypertension usually responds to sodium restriction, and control of body volume with dialysis. If renal function is sufficient, furosemide can be useful.

Hypertension that does not respond to a reduction in body volume is often associated with excess renin production. Excess sympathetic activity may also contribute. Vasoconstrictors such as endothelin, antidiuretic hormone (ADH or vasopressin), norepinephrine (noradrenaline), or a deficiency of the vasodilator nitric oxide might also play a role in this hypertension. If blood pressure cannot be controlled with angiotensin-converting enzyme inhibitors, vasodilators, or β blockers, nephrectomy is sometimes helpful. However, renal artery stenosis should be excluded as a cause of the hypertension, because it is often treatable by balloon angioplasty.

Dehydration
A loss of renal function usually causes sodium and water retention as a result of nephron loss. However, some patients preserve some filtration, but lose tubular function, and so they excrete a very dilute urine which can lead to dehydration.

Skin
Itch is the most common skin complaint. It often arises with secondary or tertiary hyperparathyroidism and may result from calcium phosphate deposition in the tissues. Itch can be helped by the control of phosphate levels and by creams that prevent dry skin. Uremic frost is the precipitation of urea crystals on the skin and happens only in severe uremia. Skin pigmentation can occur and anemia can cause pallor.

Gastrointestinal
Although gastrin levels are elevated, endoscopic studies suggest that the incidence of peptic ulceration is no higher in patients with chronic renal failure than in the general population. However, symptoms of nausea, vomiting, anorexia, and heartburn are common, and there is a higher incidence of esophagitis and angiodysplasia both of which can lead to bleeding. There is also a higher incidence of pancreatitis. Taste disturbance may be associated with a urine-like smell to the breath.

Endocrine
In men, chronic renal failure can cause loss of libido, impotence, and reduced sperm count and activity. In women, there is often loss of libido, reduced ovulation, and infertility. Abnormal growth hormone cycles contribute to growth retardation in children and loss of muscle mass in adults.

Neurologic and psychiatric
Untreated renal failure can cause fatigue, diminished consciousness, and even coma, often with signs of neurologic irritation (including tremor, asterixis, agitation, meningism, increased muscle tone with myoclonus, ankle clonus, hyperreflexia, extensor plantars, and ultimately seizures). Na^+/K^+ ATPase activity is impaired in uremia and there are parathyroid hormone (PTH)-dependent changes in membrane calcium transport which may contribute to abnormal neurotransmission.

Peripheral neuropathies can occur. The typical presentation is of a distal sensorimotor neuropathy, with glove and stocking sensory loss and distal muscle weakness and wasting. This is usually symmetrical, but can be an isolated mononeuropathy and can affect the cranial nerves. Autonomic neuropathy can also occur. Myopathy can be caused by vitamin D deficiency, hypocalcemia, hypophosphatemia, and excess PTH. Sleep disorder is common. Restless legs or muscle cramps also occur and sometimes respond to quinine sulfate. Psychiatric disturbances including depression and anxiety are common and there is an increased risk of suicide.

Immunologic
Immunologic function is impaired in chronic renal failure and infection is common. Uremia suppresses the function of most immune cells and dialysis itself can inappropriately activate immune effectors, such as complement.

Lipids
Hyperlipidemia is common, especially hypertriglyceridemia resulting from decreased triglyceride catabolism. Lipid levels are higher in patients on peritoneal dialysis than those on hemodialysis, probably as a result of the loss of regulatory plasma proteins such as apolipoprotein A-1 across the peritoneal membranes.

Cardiac disease
Pericarditis can occur and is more likely if urea or phosphate levels are high or there is severe secondary hyperparathyroidism. Fluid overload and hypertension can cause left ventricular hypertrophy or a dilated cardiomyopathy. A large arteriovenous dialysis fistula can use up a considerable proportion of cardiac output, reducing the available cardiac output for the rest of the body.

Conservative management of chronic renal failure
Management involves dietary restriction of potassium, phosphate, sodium, and water intake to avoid hyperkalemia, bone disease, and hypervolemia. Mild sustained hypervolemia can cause hypertension leading to vascular disease and left ventricular hypertrophy. Severe hypervolemia causes pulmonary edema. Blood pressure that cannot be controlled by strict fluid balance should be treated with angiotensin-converting enzyme inhibitors, β blockers, or vasodilators. Anemia should be treated with erythropoietin, after ensuring that there is no gastrointestinal or excessive menstrual blood loss and that iron, folate, and vitamin B_{12} levels are adequate. Bone disease is treated by reducing phosphate intake, taking phosphate-binding calcium salts with meals and taking vitamin D as either 1-hydroxy-vitamin D_3 or 1,25-dihydroxy-vitamin D_3.

43 Treatment of renal failure with dialysis

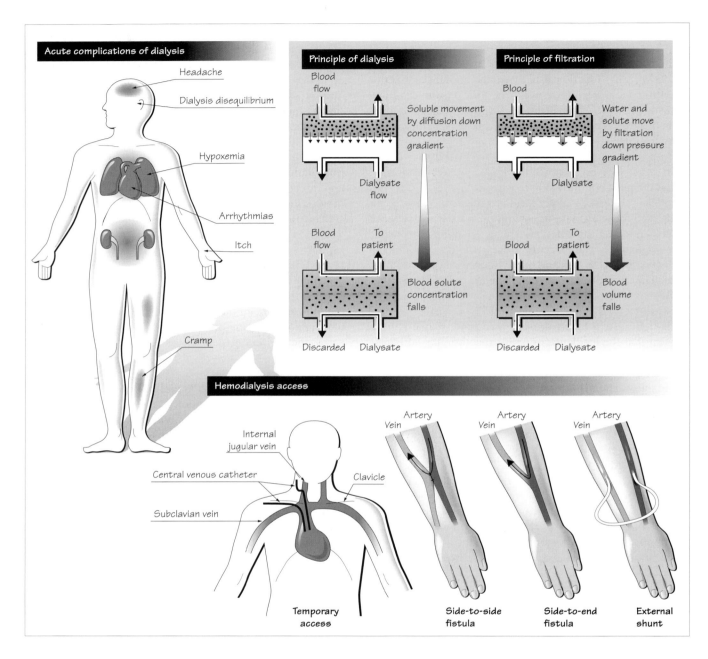

Acute complications of dialysis

- Headache
- Dialysis disequilibrium
- Hypoxemia
- Arrhythmias
- Itch
- Cramp

Principle of dialysis

Blood flow → Soluble movement by diffusion down concentration gradient → Dialysate flow

Blood flow → To patient

Blood solute concentration falls

Discarded   Dialysate

Principle of filtration

Blood → Water and solute move by filtration down pressure gradient → Dialysate

Blood → To patient

Blood volume falls

Discarded   Dialysate

Hemodialysis access

- Internal jugular vein
- Central venous catheter
- Subclavian vein
- Clavicle

Temporary access

Artery / Vein — Side-to-side fistula

Artery / Vein — Side-to-end fistula

Artery / Vein — External shunt

End-stage renal failure results from progressive chronic renal impairment or unrecovered acute renal failure. Without renal replacement therapy, death from metabolic derangement follows rapidly. Transplantation is the best treatment, but because there is a shortage of organs the initial therapy is usually dialysis, while patients wait for a transplant. Dialysis is started to treat or to prevent life-threatening hyperkalemia, acidosis, or hypervolemic pulmonary edema, or to treat complications of chronic renal failure such as pericarditis, neuropathy, seizures, and coma. The number of patients on renal replacement therapy has progressively risen since dialysis began, because more older and sicker patients can now be safely dialyzed.

Hemodialysis

Modern renal replacement uses dialysis to remove unwanted solutes by diffusion and hemofiltration to remove water which carries with it unwanted soluble substances.

The principle of dialysis

If blood is separated from a suitable fluid by a semipermeable membrane, electrolytes and other substances diffuse across the membrane until equilibrium is reached. In hemodialysis, a synthetic membrane is used, whereas in peritonal dialysis, the peritoneal membrane is used.

The principle of hemofiltration

If the blood is at a higher hydrostatic pressure than the fluid, water is forced through the membrane by ultrafiltration, carrying with it dissolved electrolytes and other substances. A high osmotic pressure can also be used to move water and dissolved substances across a semipermeable membrane. Hemofiltration is similar to glomerular filtration.

Practical aspects of hemodialysis

In hemodialysis, blood is pumped past one side of a semipermeable membrane while dialysate fluid is pumped past the other side in the opposite direction. The membranes are usually arranged within a cartridge as hollow fibers. The amount of fluid removed by ultrafiltration is controlled by altering the hydrostatic pressure of the blood compared with that of the dialysate fluid. The dialysate fluid is made up of the essential constituents of plasma—sodium, potassium, chloride, calcium, magnesium, glucose—and a buffer such as acetate, lactate, or bicarbonate. The blood and the dialysate equilibrate across the membrane. Plasma composition can therefore be controlled by altering the dialysate composition. The concentration of potassium in the dialysate is usually lower than that in the plasma to promote potassium movement out of the blood. Heparin is used in the dialysis circuit to prevent clotting. In patients at risk of bleeding, prostacyclin can be used for this, although this can cause hypotension by vasodilation.

Buffers in hemodialysis

Lactate and acetate are metabolized by the liver to produce bicarbonate. However, until this occurs, the removal of bicarbonate by dialysis lowers the $P\text{CO}_2$ and this can inhibit ventilation, contributing to hypoxemia. Acetate is also a vasodilator and so can cause hypotension. Bicarbonate is the preferred base, but it precipitates with calcium or magnesium and must be made up just before dialysis. It is useful in unstable patients and when liver disease impairs lactate or acetate metabolism.

Dialysis access

Hemodialysis ideally requires two points of access to the circulation: one to remove blood and one to return it from the dialyzer. In the short term, this can be achieved with a large-bore dual-lumen central venous catheter. This can be tunneled through the skin to reduce the risk of infection.

However, for long-term access, an artificial arteriovenous fistula is usually created in the arm by joining the radial or brachial artery to a vein, in a side-to-side or side-to-end manner. Over several months, the fistula dilates and the high flow through it allows two large-bore needles to be placed in it for dialysis. A fistula can also be constructed by joining the artery and vein with a synthetic polytetrafluoroethylene (Goretex) graft. Occasionally, an external shunt is used to join the artery to the vein. In renal patients, intravenous lines should always be sited on the back of the hand, rather than on the arm, to avoid damage to arm veins that may be needed later for fistula construction.

Acute complications of hemodialysis

Movement of blood out of the circulation into the dialysis circuit can cause *hypotension*. Over-aggressive initial dialysis can cause *dialysis disequilibrium*, as a result of the osmotic changes in the brain as the plasma urea falls. The effects range from nausea and headache to seizures and coma. *Headache* during dialysis can also result from the vasodilatory effect of acetate. *Itch* during or after hemodialysis may reflect the itch of chronic renal failure, exacerbated by histamine release caused by a mild allergic reaction to the dialysis membrane. Rarely, exposure of blood to the dialysis membrane can cause a more generalized allergic response, which is less likely with expensive biocompatible membranes. *Cramps* on dialysis probably reflect electrolyte shifts across muscle membranes. *Hypoxemia* during dialysis may reflect hypoventilation caused by the removal of bicarbonate or pulmonary shunting as a result of vasomotor changes that are induced by substances activated by the dialysis membrane. Reducing potassium levels excessively causes *hypokalemia* and dysrhythmias. Problems in the dialysis circuit can cause *air embolism* which should be treated by placing the patient head down on their left side with 100% oxygen.

Chronic complications of hemodialysis

The most common problems involve access and include fistula thrombosis and aneurysm formation and infection, especially with synthetic grafts or temporary central venous access. Systemic infection can be introduced at the access site or acquired from the dialysis circuit. Transmission of blood-borne infections such as viral hepatitis and HIV infection is a potential hazard. With long-term dialysis, deposition of dialysis amyloid protein containing β_2-microglobulin can cause carpal tunnel syndrome and a destructive arthropathy with cystic bone lesions. Phosphate-binding compounds that contain aluminum and aluminum contamination of dialysate fluid causes aluminum toxicity with dementia, myoclonus, seizures, and bone disease. The condition improves with deferoxamine (desferrioxamine) treatment.

Peritoneal dialysis and continuous hemofiltration

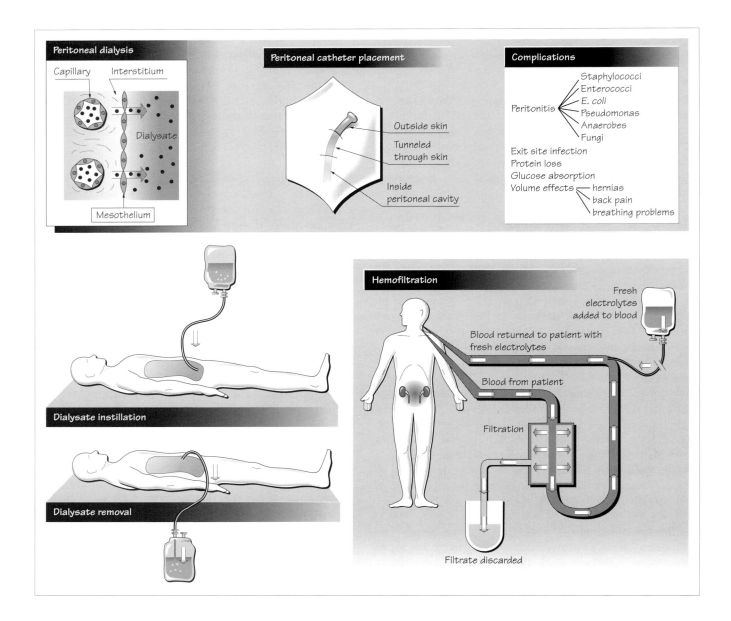

Peritoneal dialysis

Peritoneal dialysis relies on the movement of solutes and water across the semipermeable peritoneal membrane. The membrane consists of three layers: the mesothelium, the interstitium, and the peritoneal capillary wall. Water moves from plasma to a dialysate solution with a high glucose content by osmosis. Solutes move with the water and also diffuse into the dialysate. Peritoneal dialysis is slower than hemodialysis, so hypotension, hypoxia, dysrhythmias, and disequilibrium are uncommon. Peritoneal dialysis may clear some uremic toxins better than hemodialysis and

it is associated with less bone disease, anemia, and hypertension.

Technical aspects of peritoneal dialysis

Soft Silastic catheters are usually tunneled through the skin and placed in the peritoneal cavity to provide permanent access to the peritoneal cavity. Formerly, semirigid catheters were used for short-term acute dialysis. Bags of sterile dialysate are attached to the peritoneal catheter and drained into the peritoneal cavity by gravity. The catheter is clamped with the empty bag connected and, when the dialysis is finished, the catheter is unclamped and the fluid drained by gravity into the bag, which is then disconnected and discarded. The technique is termed **continuous ambulatory peritoneal dialysis (CAPD)** because patients can go about their normal daily activities with the fluid in the abdomen. Patients usually instill a fresh 2L of dialysate every 4h. It is common to instill a 'strong' bag of high osmotic strength overnight to remove water. Around three to four 'exchanges' are used each day. **Intermittent peritoneal dialysis** is a less common approach. A machine pumps fresh fluid into the peritoneal cavity every 20min for a 24- to 48-h period.

With both methods, any residual renal function contributes significantly to the overall efficiency of the dialysis. Peritoneal dialysis must start with small volumes and only when the catheter is secure and uninfected. Peritoneal dialysis may not be possible if abdominal surgery or sepsis has caused fibrosis, adhesions, or loss of a peritoneal surface area suitable for dialysis.

Complications of peritoneal dialysis
Infection
The major problem is infection causing peritonitis. Most infection comes from skin-derived Gram-positive staphylococci or gut-derived Gram-negative organisms such as *Escherichia coli*, or rarely anaerobic organisms or fungi. Infection can cause fever, abdominal pain, and tenderness. Dialysate fluid is cloudy when it is removed from the abdomen and contains excess white blood cells (>100 cells/mm^3 with more than 50% neutrophils). Treatment is a few fluid exchanges to wash out the peritoneum and then normal dialysis continues, but antibiotics are added to the dialysis bags or given systemically. Usually vancomycin is used to cover Gram-positive infection and an aminoglycoside, ciprofloxacin, or ceftazidime to cover Gram-negative organisms. If the infection is severe or fungal, the catheter should be removed and systemic antibiotics used. Unfortunately, repeated peritonitis can reduce the permeability of the peritoneal membrane. Infection can also occur around the catheter exit site.

Other complications
Around 5–10g of protein is lost into the dialysate fluid each day, so protein intake must compensate for this. The loss is increased during peritonitis. A significant amount of glucose is absorbed from the bags and this can be troublesome for people with diabetes and may contribute to hypertriglyceridemia. Other complications include hernias, impaired ventilatory capacity, and back pain, as a result of

the intra-abdominal pressure. β_2-Microglobulin is better cleared by peritoneal dialysis than by hemodialysis, so dialysis amyloid is very rare.

Continuous hemofiltration
With continuous hemofiltration, venous blood is pumped at a high pressure on to a highly permeable membrane to produce large volumes of ultrafiltrate, analogous to glomerular filtration. The filtrate is then discarded and replaced by an appropriate volume of a balanced electrolyte solution which is added back to the blood. This solution contains sodium, potassium, chloride, calcium, magnesium, and a buffer such as acetate, lactate, or bicarbonate. The big advantage of the technique over dialysis is that it is slow and continuous, which avoids the rapid solute changes of dialysis. The technique is suitable for hemodynamically unstable patients with acute renal failure and is easily performed through a dual-lumen central venous catheter. As with hemodialysis, blood is anticoagulated with heparin or prostacyclin. Continuous arteriovenous hemofiltration is an older method which uses the patient's arterial blood pressure as the driving force for filtration.

Special related procedures
Plasma exchange
Plasma exchange removes antibodies and other large immunologically active molecules from plasma in order to treat immune-mediated diseases. Very highly permeable membranes are used to filter plasma away from the blood cells and, as in hemofiltration, the filtrate is discarded and replaced by a new solution. The replacement fluid must also contain protein such as albumin and electrolytes. Clotting factors are removed by the process and fresh frozen plasma is usually given to reduce the risk of bleeding. Centrifugation can be used to separate plasma from blood cells in a process known as centrifugal apheresis.

Hemoperfusion
Hemoperfusion is used to remove poisons from the blood. In hemoperfusion, blood is pumped through a cartridge containing activated charcoal which is coated with a biocompatible substance; it is then returned to the patient. The charcoal binds most drugs and poisons, but newer polymers and resins are being developed to bind specific substances. Columns containing specific antigens can be used to bind and remove specific antibodies against the antigen. Immunoadsorption has been used before transplantation to remove alloantibodies from patients who have antibodies against donor molecules.

45 Renal transplantation

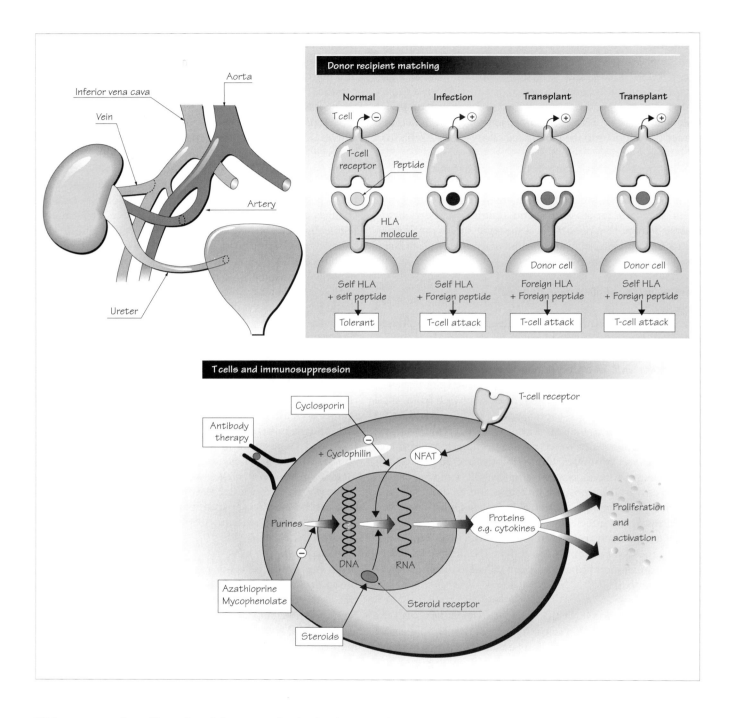

Kidneys come from live related donors or brain dead or recently deceased donors; they are implanted in the right or left iliac fossa. The renal artery is sutured to the external or internal iliac artery and the renal vein to the external iliac vein, and the ureter is implanted in the bladder wall. The immune system attacks foreign material, including trans-planted organs. Humans have many polymorphic genes which cause differences between individuals, identifying a transplant as foreign. For example, to avoid immediate anti-body attack, the donor organ and the recipient must have compatible blood types.

The **human leukocyte antigens (HLAs)** are highly polymorphic. HLA mismatches, particularly in HLA-A, HLA-B, or HLA-DR molecules between the transplant organ and the recipient, substantially increase the risk of rejection and are avoided if possible. HLA molecules bind peptide fragments of protein antigens in a groove on their surface for recognition by T lymphocytes. Normally, peptides from self-proteins are bound and recognized as self by T cells. During infection, pathogen-derived peptides are bound which triggers an immune attack. During unmatched transplantation, T cells encounter foreign HLA molecules; these, regardless of the bound peptide, are seen as foreign and trigger an immune attack. Even matched HLA molecules in a transplant organ can bind peptides from other unmatched polymorphic molecules and provoke an immune attack.

Immunosuppression

Immunosuppression inhibits immune responses and reduces the chance of rejection, but increases the risk of infection and tumors.

Steroids such as the glucocorticoids prednisolone and methylprednisolone bind steroid receptors, inhibiting gene transcription and immunologic function in T cells, macrophages, and neutrophils. *Side effects* include infection, peptic ulceration, osteoporosis, hypertension, hyperglycemia, obesity, mood swings, poor wound healing, cataracts, and suppression of adrenal glucocorticoid production.

Cyclosporin forms a complex with cyclophilin, which inhibits calcineurin. Calcineurin normally dephosphorylates the transcription factor NF-AT, allowing it to enter the nucleus. In the nucleus, NF-AT promotes expression of cytokines, especially interleukin-2 (IL-2) which is required for T-cell activation. Cyclosporin therefore inhibits IL-2 synthesis and T-cell activation. *Side effects* include nephrotoxicity, hyperkalemia, hypomagnesemia, hypertension, heptatotoxicity, gum hyperplasia, and hirsutism. Acute nephrotoxicity results from renal vasoconstriction. Chronic nephrotoxicity is caused by glomerular ischemia and interstitial fibrosis. Plasma cyclosporin levels must be monitored. Drugs that induce hepatic cytochrome P450 activity lower the drug level.

Azathioprine is metabolized to 6-mercaptopurine, which inhibits purine metabolism, nucleic acid synthesis, and cell proliferation, especially in lymphocytes and neutrophils. *Side effects* include infection, pancreatitis, and bone marrow depression with neutropenia and sometimes megaloblastic anemia and thrombocytopenia. Allopurinol can cause toxic 6-mercaptopurine levels by inhibiting xanthine oxidase, the enzyme that degrades it.

Mycophenolate inhibits inosine monophosphate dehydrogenase—an enzyme required for nucleic acid synthesis. Similar to azathioprine, it inhibits B- and T-cell function. *Side effects* include esophagitis, gastritis, and diarrhea, but not bone marrow suppression.

Tacrolimus and rapamycin bind to immunophilins such as cyclophilin. Tacrolimus (FK506) has a similar effect to cyclosporin and also causes nephrotoxicity and hypertension. Rapamycin inhibits signaling through the IL-2 receptor, blocks the progression of T cells through the cell cycle, and inhibits B cells.

Antibody therapy. Polyclonal horse or rabbit antibodies against human white blood cells can be used for immunosuppression at the time of transplantation. Monoclonal antibodies against surface molecules on T cells have a similar role.

Future transplantation strategies. Ideally, immunosuppression would inhibit only the immune response against the transplanted organ, leaving other responses intact. Alternatively, tolerance to the organ could be induced before transplantation. Genetically modified pigs are being developed that are less immunogenic than normal pig tissues.

Complications of transplantation
Early complications of transplantation

Poor renal function may indicate acute rejection, cyclosporin toxicity, or acute tubular necrosis caused by ischemia before the kidney was revascularized. Biopsy of the transplanted organ may distinguish these possibilities. Pre- and postrenal problems can also arise. **Cellular rejection** is a cell-mediated process and is treated with drugs or antibody therapy. **Vascular rejection** is more aggressive and often antibody mediated. There is usually vessel damage and plasma exchange is used to remove the antibodies. **Cytomegalovirus infection** can cause fever, retinopathy, hepatitis, enteritis, pneumonitis, and thrombocytopenia. Treatment is with gancyclovir or foscarnet. **Post-transplant lymphoproliferative disease** is a lymphoma-like disease caused by the Epstein–Barr virus early after transplantation. It may respond to withdrawal of immunosuppression.

Chronic complications of transplantation

Loss of renal function as a result of both immune and non-immune mechanisms is termed chronic rejection. Contributing factors include immunologic rejection, cyclosporin nephrotoxicity, hypertension, and recurrent disease (especially focal segmental glomerulosclerosis, membranoproliferative nephropathy, and IgA nephropathy). **Hypertension** may result from steroid use, cyclosporin-induced vasoconstriction, renin secretion by the native kidneys, or renal artery stenosis of the transplanted organ. **Hyperlipidemia** is common with steroid or cyclosporin therapy. Steroids also cause generalized **osteoporosis** and osteonecrosis of the femoral head. High parathyroid hormone (PTH) levels may cause phosphaturia requiring phosphate supplements and sometimes hypercalcemia. **Skin cancer** is a common late complication and the incidence is increased by sun exposure.

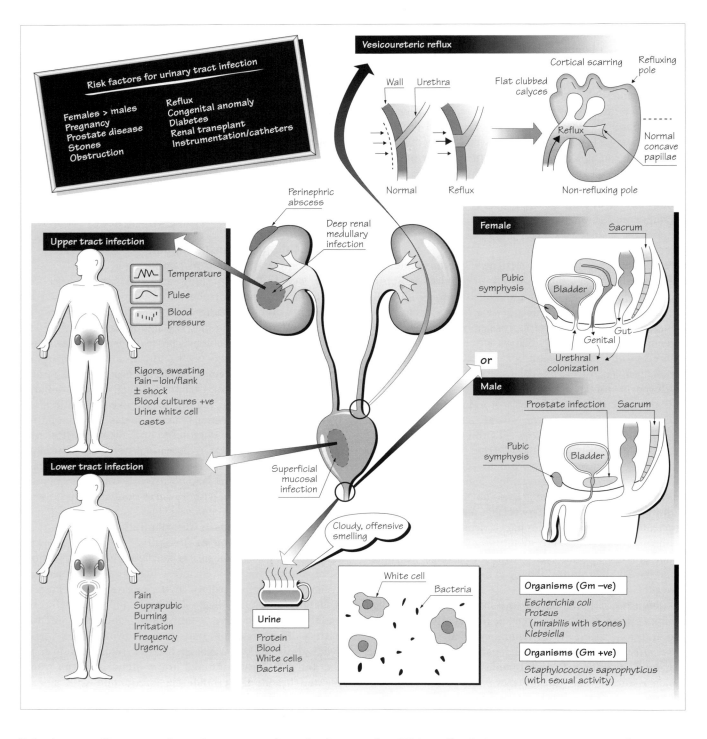

Infection usually enters the urinary tract through the urethra, but blood-borne infection can deposit in the kidney. Urinary tract infection is diagnosed when there are >100000 organisms of the same bacterial species per mL of urine. White cell tubular casts suggest upper urinary tract infection.

Lower urinary tract infection is restricted to the bladder and urethra. It usually involves only the *superficial* mucosa and has no long-term effects. **Upper urinary tract infection**, affecting the kidney or ureters, involves the *deep* renal medullary tissue and can permanently damage the kidney.

Factors predisposing to urinary tract infection

Urinary tract infection is more common in women than in men and peaks during the child-bearing years. The short female urethra provides easy bladder access for organisms that colonize the perineum from the bowel and genital tract. During voiding, the short urethra may also cause turbulence and back-flow. In women, sexual activity, especially initially or with a new partner, is associated with infection, because bacteria in perineal secretions may be massaged up the urethra. Voiding before and after sexual activity reduces infection. During pregnancy, endocrine changes, especially the high progesterone level, cause dilation and reduce the tone of the ureters, which in turn increases the risk of upper tract infection. Static urine above an obstruction or caused by incomplete bladder emptying is at risk of infection. Infection can also spread from a focus such as a chronically infected prostate gland or a urinary stone (typically with *Proteus mirabilis*). Instrumentation or catheterization of the urinary tract can introduce infection and indwelling catheters pose a continued risk of infection. Diabetes and immunosuppression, especially in renal transplant recipients, predispose to urinary infection. A single urinary infection in a woman of child-bearing age requires no investigation. In other groups, or women with recurrent or severe infection, a predisposing condition should be sought. Useful investigations include plain radiography and ultrasonography to exclude stones, obstruction, and anatomical anomalies. In men, the prostate must be assessed by rectal examination.

Clinical syndromes

Asymptotic bacteriuria

Routine screening detects asymptomatic bacteriuria in around 5% of women, especially during pregnancy. Around 30% progress to symptomatic infection within a year. In pregnancy, this is upper tract infection, so pregnant women are screened and treated to prevent renal damage. In pregnancy nitrofurantoin, ampicillin, cephalosporins, or nalidixic acid are used. Men with asymptomatic bacteriuria usually have prostatic disease or obstructive uropathy.

Acute, uncomplicated, lower urinary tract infection

This is common and affects mainly women of child-bearing age. The symptoms are of urethritis (burning or stinging on passing urine) and of cystitis or bladder inflammation (lower abdominal pain or discomfort, and urinary frequency and urgency). Small volumes of urine may be passed frequently and nocturia is common. The urine may be cloudy and offensive smelling. Hematuria can occur. The condition is usually self-limiting if a high urine flow is maintained by a good fluid intake. Antibiotics provide symptomatic relief and reduce the chance of chronic infection. The usual organisms are Gram-negative *Escherichia coli*, *Klebsiella* and *Proteus* species. *Staphylococcus saprophyticus* is also common in sexually active young women. Treatment for 1–5 days with the common antibiotics ampicillin, cephalosporins, trimethoprim, and the sulfonamides is usually adequate.

Recurrent urinary tract infection

This term refers to repeated episodes of symptomatic infection, separated by symptom-free periods, which are often simply periods of asymptomatic infection. A predisposing risk factor should be sought, although in women it is uncommon to find one. Failure to eradicate the organism from deep upper tract infection sites leads to relapse and up to 6 weeks of antibiotics may be necessary. In superficial lower tract infection, organisms are easily eradicated and relapse usually represents reinfection.

Acute pyelonephritis

Typically, there is loin pain, fever, flank tenderness, and bacteremia. Rigors can occur with malaise and vomiting. The kidney may be palpable and tender. Infection is mainly in the renal medulla with white cell infiltration around the tubules. Urine cultures and often blood cultures are positive and there may be white cell casts in the urine.

Acute complicated urinary tract infection

This term refers to infection with a predisposing risk factor such as a stone or obstruction. Antibiotics are usually only effective if the complicating factor is treated.

Vesico-ureteric reflux in children

Any childhood urinary tract infection must be investigated. The most important risk factor is vesicoureteric reflux caused by an abnormal entrance of the ureter into the bladder. During voiding, bladder wall contraction normally closes the ureteric orifice and the angle of the ureter in the bladder wall creates a flap valve preventing reflux. However, if the ureter does not pass diagonally through the bladder wall and the orifice is enlarged, voiding causes reflux up the ureter and into the renal pelvis. Within the renal pelvis, there may be intrarenal reflux into the medulla. The reflux usually resolves by adulthood, but most damage occurs before the age of 5 and reflux nephropathy may account for 10–15% of end-stage renal failure. The renal damage is termed chronic pyelonephritis and is diagnosed radiologically with clubbing of the renal calyces and cortical scarring. Vesicoureteric reflux is diagnosed by a micturating cystourethrogram—contrast medium is placed in the bladder via a suprapubic or urethral catheter and images are taken during voiding to see if the medium goes up the ureters.

Renal tract stones

Stone type	Percentage of patients	Visible on X-ray	Risk factors in urine	Secondary causes
Calcium	80	Yes	$Ca^{2+}\uparrow$ Oxalate$\uparrow$ Citrate$\downarrow$ Volume$\downarrow$	$Ca^{2+}\uparrow$ — Malignancy / Sarcoidosis / Vitamin D intake Oxalate$\uparrow$ — Primary hyperoxaluria type 1 / Ileal disease Citrate$\downarrow$ — Distal renal tubular acidosis
Urate	10	No	Urate$\uparrow$ pH$\downarrow$ Volume$\downarrow$	With blood urate$\uparrow$ — Cell death / Inborn metabolic defects / Gout With blood urate normal — probenicid Acid urine—gut disease
Cystine	2	Weakly	Cystine$\uparrow$	Cystinuria
Infection	5	Yes	pH$\uparrow$ infection	Urea-splitting bacteria — Proteus
Others	3			Xanthinuria Drugs Metabolic defects

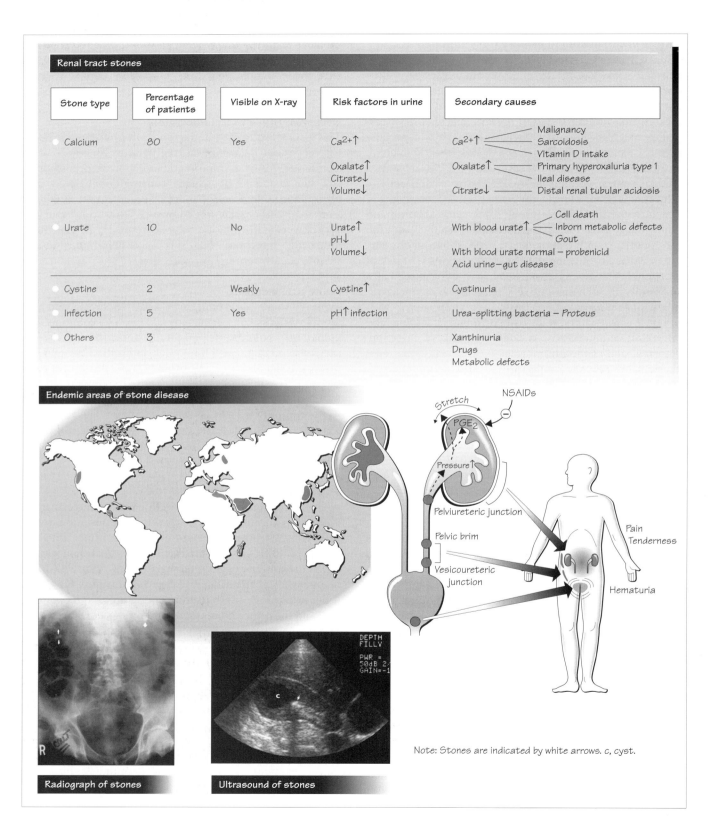

Endemic areas of stone disease

NSAIDs

Stretch

PGE_2

Pressure$\uparrow$

Pelviureteric junction

Pelvic brim

Vesicoureteric junction

Pain
Tenderness

Hematuria

Radiograph of stones

Ultrasound of stones

DEPTH
FILLV
PWR =
50dB 2/
GAIN=-1

Note: Stones are indicated by white arrows. c, cyst.

Urinary stasis, infection, and indwelling catheters all promote stone formation. Stones form if stone-forming substances reach high enough concentrations to crystallize out of solution. However, debris or other crystals can cause crystal growth at lower concentrations. Urinary citrate inhibits stone formation by forming soluble complexes with calcium. Rare renal chloride channel mutations can cause stones (see Chapter 16). **Nephrocalcinosis** describes diffuse renal calcium deposition, mainly in the medulla. Causes include hyperparathyroidism, distal renal tubular acidosis, and medullary sponge kidney.

Clinical presentation

Stones can cause recurrent infection, renal impairment, or hematuria. Acute obstruction causes renal colic with intense flank pain, often radiating to the groin, and sometimes nausea, vomiting, abdominal discomfort, dysuria, renal tenderness, and hematuria. Obstruction stretches the renal capsule, causing severe pain with increased renal prostaglandin E_2 production. If there is good renal function, non-steroidal anti-inflammatory drugs are, therefore, effective analgesics. Stones can lodge in the ureter at the pelvi-ureteric junction, at the pelvic brim, or at the ureterovesical junction. The renal pelvis refers pain to the loin and back, the lower ureter to the testis or labium majus, and the lowest pelvic part of the ureter to the tip of the penis or perineum. Bladder stones can halt urine flow suddenly, with penile or perineal pain which may be relieved by lying down.

Calcium stones

These are the most common type and contain calcium oxalate, calcium phosphate, or both. Predisposing factors are low urine volume, high urine calcium, high urine oxalate, and a low urine citrate level. **Hypercalciuria** occurs in 65% of patients who have stones. It is usually idiopathic and associated with increased intestinal calcium absorption, obesity, and hypertension. Fluid intake should be increased and calcium, sodium, and animal protein intake decreased. Thiazides inhibit calcium excretion and potassium or citrate levels are corrected with potassium citrate. Excess calcium intake or any cause of hypercalcemia can cause hypercalciuria, especially primary hyperparathyroidism. Excess dietary sodium raises urine calcium levels by lowering proximal tubule sodium reabsorption and co-transport of calcium. Animal protein intake also increases urine calcium levels. **Oxalate** is a metabolic end-product excreted in the urine. Hyperoxaluria can result from excess dietary intake, excess colonic absorption with ileal disease or from inborn errors of metabolism. **Hypocitraturia** can be idiopathic or result from distal renal tubular acidosis, which causes excess mitochondrial metabolism of citrate.

Urate stones

Sodium urate is relatively insoluble at acid pH. Most cases are *idiopathic* with normal blood and urine urate levels, but often with acidic urine. Treatment involves reducing the dietary purine intake, increasing the urine volume, and urine alkalinization with sodium bicarbonate or potassium citrate. Allopurinol inhibits urate production. *Secondary* causes include inborn errors of purine metabolism and rapid cell turnover or death, especially during cancer chemotherapy. Good hydration and sometimes alkalinization provide prophylaxis. Acid urine is produced when there is loss of alkaline bowel contents as a result of diarrhea, an ileostomy, or laxative abuse.

Cystine stones

An autosomal recessive defect in the renal dibasic amino acid transporter reduces tubular cystine reabsorption, causing *cystinuria*. Cystine is relatively insoluble especially at acid pH. Prophylaxis consists of a good fluid intake and alkalinization with sodium bicarbonate. Dimethylcysteine (D-pencillamine) can be used to cleave cystine into soluble components.

Infection stones

These are often large staghorn calculi containing magnesium ammonium phosphate and calcium phosphate. Infection, usually with *Proteus* species, produces urease which splits urea to produce ammonium ions. The rise in pH promotes calcium phosphate crystallization and the ammonium crystallizes with magnesium and phosphate. Treatment involves removal of the stones, antibiotics to eradicate infection, and screening for an underlying stone-forming predisposition.

Acute investigation and treatment

Plain radiography may show radio-opaque stones. Ultrasonography detects all stone types. Exclude urinary infection and check renal function. Stones less than 6 mm in diameter usually pass spontaneously, but stones more than 1 cm will not. Obstruction must be relieved. Stones can be removed by extracorporeal shock wave lithotripsy (ESWL), endoscopically, percutaneously, or by conventional surgery. ESWL aims shock waves at the stone through the skin, but can be complicated by bleeding and sepsis.

Investigation of patients with stones

History and clinical examination should exclude bowel disease, diarrhea, and the use of antacids and diuretics. Diet should be assessed for fluid, protein, sodium, calcium, oxalate, purine, and vitamin D intake and a family history taken. Stones should be analyzed to determine their constituents. Baseline investigations include urinalysis, serum calcium, phosphate, urate, creatinine, and urea. Recurrent stone formation merits 24-h urine collections for volume, osmolality, calcium, phosphate, oxalate, citrate, urate, sodium creatinine, pH, as well as serum sodium, potassium, chloride, and bicarbonate.

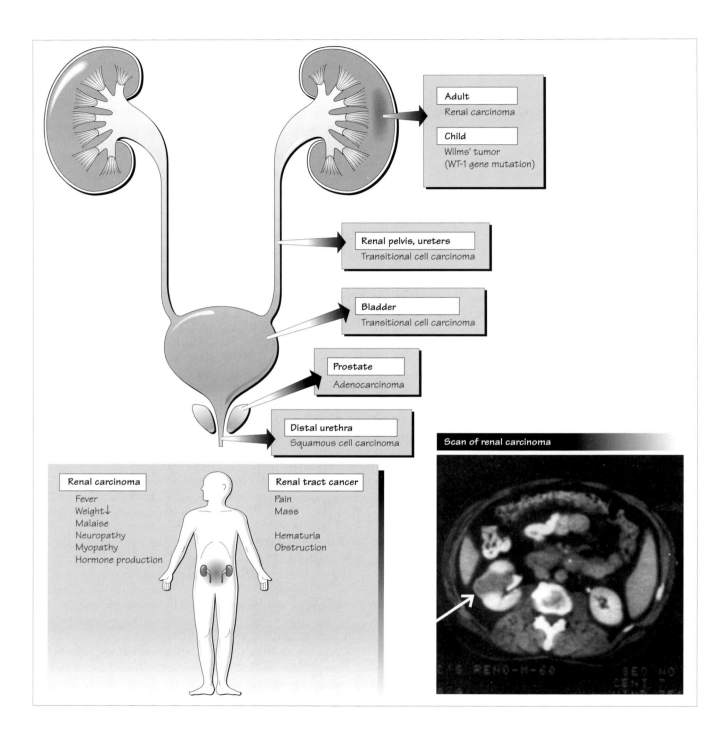

Scan of renal carcinoma

Tumors at different sites along the renal tract can cause hematuria or altered urinary flow.

Renal tumors in adults

Adult renal cancer usually arises in the proximal tubules and is known as renal carcinoma, renal cell carcinoma, or hypernephroma. It accounts for about 2% of adult malignancies. Most patients are over 50 years of age; the risk is increased in men and people who smoke. The tumor spreads locally or via the lymphatics to the renal hilum, retroperitoneum, and para-aortic nodes. It often invades the renal veins and inferior vena cava. Blockage of the right testicular vein, which drains into the inferior vena cava, causes a right-sided varicocele. The left testicular vein drains into the left renal vein and left renal vein occlusion causes a left-sided varicocele. Metastases typically arise in the lung, liver, bones, and brain.

The usual **presentation** is hematuria, but there may be loin, back, or abdominal pain. As the blood is from high in the renal tract, hematuria is usually frank and uniform throughout the stream. On examination, there may be an abdominal mass, groin or neck lymphadenopathy, skin metastases, or a large liver or spleen. Systemic effects are common, including weight loss, night sweats, fever, anemia, nausea, malaise, polyneuritis, and myositis. Renal tumors can produce excess hormones such as erythropoietin, renin, or PTH-related protein (PTHrP) causing erythrocytosis, hypertension, or hypercalcemia, respectively. **Investigation** includes urinalysis and cytology, imaging by ultrasonography, computed tomography, or magnetic resonance imaging. Treatment is surgical removal of the tumor and often the entire kidney. Immunotherapy with interferon-α and interleukin-2 can be of benefit.

Secondary renal tumors can arise from lung or breast tumors, melanomas, or lymphomas. Von Hippel–Lindau disease is an autosomal dominant condition caused by mutations in a gene on chromosome 3. It causes tumors in the kidneys, eyes, central nervous system, gonads, adrenals, and pancreas.

Wilms' tumor in children

This accounts for 8% of childhood cancers with a peak incidence at 2–3 years of age. It occurs alone or as part of a syndrome such as the WAGR syndrome (**W**ilms' tumor, **a**niridia, **g**enitourinary malformations, learning disorder/mental **r**etardation). Presentation is usually with an abdominal mass, although hematuria, pain, or fever can occur. A cure is usually achieved with nephrectomy and chemotherapy. Wilms' tumor is caused by mutations in the *WT-1* gene on chromosome 11.

Urothelial tumors

The renal tract is lined by transitional epithelium from the tips of the renal papillae to the proximal urethra, and by squamous epithelium in the distal urethra. Most transitional epithelial tumors arise in the bladder. Tumor in the urethra is uncommon and can be caused by spread of bladder cancers or primary urethral squamous cell carcinomas, particularly after chronic inflammation.

Bladder cancer

Bladder cancer has a peak incidence around 65 years of age. Risk factors include smoking, chronic bladder inflammation (especially from schistosomiasis infection), and exposure to industrial toxins from the dye industry. Tumors are usually transitional cell tumors, but 5% are squamous cell tumors, which usually follow chronic inflammation. Tumors are staged according to the extent of invasion through the bladder wall. There may be local spread into the pelvis, but distant metastasis is uncommon. The typical presentation is with painless hematuria. A bladder mass or obstructed kidney may be palpable. Investigation includes urine analysis and urine cytology, imaging using ultrasonography, computed tomography, magnetic resonance imaging, and cystoscopy and if necessary examination under anesthesia. Contrast studies may show a filling defect. Sterile pyuria can occur—pus cells such as polymorphonuclear leukocytes in the absence of infection.

Superficial bladder tumors can be resected endoscopically followed by repeated cystoscopic surveillance to detect recurrence. Deeper tumors may require total cystectomy, sometimes with removal of other pelvic contents. Radiotherapy or chemotherapy may be added. Carcinoma *in situ* describes malignant change over most of the surface epithelium. It causes similar symptoms to cystitis, and is treated with intravesical chemotherapy or intravesical BCG (bacille Calmette–Guérin) to trigger inflammation and promote tumor regression.

Prostate cancer

Prostate cancer is the third most common cancer in men. Most cancers are adenocarcinomas arising in the posterior outer zone of the prostate. They initially spread by local invasion and then involve pelvic lymph nodes, metastasizing to bone, especially the lumbar spine and pelvis, and less commonly to the lung and liver. Bone metastases are typically denser than normal bone tissue.

Presentation is usually with the symptoms of bladder outflow obstruction such as hesitancy, poor stream, terminal dribbling, frequency, nocturia, urinary retention, or obstruction. The tumor is usually hard and irregular on rectal examination. The main differential diagnosis is benign prostatic hypertrophy. Prostatic cells secrete prostate-specific antigen (PSA) and acid phosphatase, which are usually elevated in the presence of a tumor. Transrectal ultrasonography can be used to identify and biopsy tumors. Early tumors are treated with transurethral resection of the prostate (TURP) and regular follow-up. Advanced tumors may require radical prostatectomy and radiotherapy. Tumor growth may be promoted by testosterone. Hormonal therapy of metastatic disease includes orchidectomy, synthetic estrogens, androgen receptor antagonists such as cyproterone acetate or flutamide, and gonadotropin-releasing hormone analogues such as buserelin.

For each case, read the clinical section first and try to assemble some ideas about what the problem might be. This is how the clinician would have to approach the problem in real life. Then look at the investigations and see whether or not your ideas are confirmed and answer the questions. Don't look at the explanatory answers until you have answered the questions yourself.

Case 1: A 10-year-old with generalized swelling

A 10-year-old boy presented with generalized swelling. This had been present for 4 days and included swollen ankles and puffiness of the face. It started a few days after he had had a mild cold with a runny nose. His only past medical history was of mild eczema. On examination, there were no abnormalities apart from the swelling which included pitting edema around both ankles.

Urinalysis showed protein +++ and a 24-h urine collection contained 10 g protein/24 h. His serum creatinine was normal at 60 μmol/L (0.7 mg/dL), but his serum albumin was low at 20 g/L (2.0 g/dL).
- What clinical syndrome does he have?
- What is the probable pathologic diagnosis?
- What is the usual treatment?

Case 2: A family history of hypertension and renal impairment

A 34-year-old man was noted on a routine employment examination to be hypertensive (BP 180/100). His father and his father's sister had both had hypertension and developed end-stage renal failure and his father had received a kidney transplant. On examination, there were large palpable kidneys bilaterally.

His serum creatinine was raised at 280 μmol/L (3.2 mg/dL).
- What is the likely diagnosis?
- What investigation would confirm the diagnosis?
- What is his prognosis?

Case 3: Colicky loin pain

A 45-year-old man presented with sudden-onset, severe, right-sided loin pain. The pain was colicky in nature. On examination he was very tender in the right loin.

Urinalysis showed blood ++. A full blood count was normal. His plasma biochemistry showed a normal plasma creatinine of 101 μmol/L (1.1 mg/dL) and normal electrolytes apart from a raised calcium of 2.7 mmol/L (10.8 mg/dL). His plasma albumin level was normal at 40 g/L (4.0 g/dL).
- What is the likely cause of the pain?

- What investigation would confirm the cause of the pain?
- Does he have a metabolic predisposition to his current problem and what might its etiology be?

Case 4: An older man with nocturia and poor urinary flow

A 72-year-old man presented with nocturia of up to eight times a night. He also complained that the flow of his urine was poor. He often had to wait for several minutes before the flow would start and, at the end of the stream, he experienced significant dribbling of urine. On examination he had a palpable enlarged bladder even though he had just voided.

His serum electrolytes were normal apart from a urea (blood urea nitrogen or BUN) of 20 mmol/L (56.0 mg/dL) and a creatinine of 240 μmol/L (2.7 mg/dL).
- What is the essential part of the clinical examination?
- Why are the plasma urea and creatinine raised?
- What blood tests might indicate the etiology of the disease?

Case 5: Postoperative confusion in a young woman

A 35-year-old woman became acutely confused and lethargic in hospital, 2 days after surgery for acute appendicitis. She had not been able to eat or drink since the operation. Her temperature was normal and she was well hydrated.

Her blood electrolytes showed a low sodium of 118 mmol/L, a normal potassium of 3.8 mmol/L, and a creatinine of 90 μmol/L (1.0 mg/dL).
- What is the most likely cause of her confusion?
- What is the probable etiology of this disorder?
- How should she be treated?

Case 6: Renal problems after vascular surgery

A 68-year-old man presented with acute severe abdominal pain. On examination he was cold, clammy, and hypotensive. Blood was taken, which showed a normal plasma creatinine of 105 μmol/L (1.2 mg/dL). He was taken immediately to the operating room, where a ruptured abdominal aortic aneurysm was identified and repaired. Two days after the operation, he was noted to be passing no urine.

His plasma creatinine was 415 μmol/L (4.7 mg/dL).
- What are the possible causes of his acute renal failure?
- What investigations might help to distinguish these possibilities?
- What problems might require urgent renal replacement therapy?

Case 7: Hypertension and renal impairment

A 65-year-old smoker presented with a left-sided stroke. He had weakness of the left arm and leg. On examination, he had a blood pressure of 180/95 and bilateral carotid bruits and bilateral abdominal bruits.

His plasma creatinine was elevated at 190 μmol/L (2.2 mg/dL).

• What could explain both his hypertension and his renal impairment?

• What investigations might be helpful in diagnosing the cause of his hypertension?

• What might happen if he was given an angiotensin-converting enzyme inhibitor?

Case 8: General malaise and itch with a pericardial rub

A 43-year-old woman presented to hospital with tiredness, itch, nausea, and general malaise. On examination, she was drowsy and pale and had a pericardial friction rub.

Her biochemical tests showed a sodium of 142 mmol/L, a potassium of 5.1 mmol/L, a calcium of 1.7 mmol/L (6.8 mg/dL), a phosphate of 3.8 mmol/L (11.7 mg/dL), and an albumin of 37 g/L (3.7 g/dL). Her plasma urea (blood urea nitrogen or BUN) was 60 mmol/L (168 mg/dL) and her plasma creatinine was 1400 μmol/L (15.8 mg/dL). Her full blood count showed a hemoglobin level of 7.1 g/dL, a white cell count of 6.2×10^9 cells/L (6.2×10^3 cells/μL) and a platelet count of 192×10^3/μL. A renal ultrasound scan showed two small unobstructed kidneys.

• Does she have acute or chronic renal failure?

• What factors contribute to the low plasma calcium level?

• Is her parathyroid hormone (PTH) level likely to be high or low?

Case 9: A young girl with thirst and rapid breathing

A 15-year-old girl presented with a history of thirst and general malaise over 2–3 weeks. On examination, she had deep rapid breathing and was dehydrated. Her pulse rate was 110 and her blood pressure was 90/70 lying and 70/50 standing.

Her urine showed glucose +++ and ketones +++ on dipstick analysis. Her blood tests showed plasma sodium 132 mmol/L, potassium 3.7 mmol/L, urea (BUN) 8 mmol/L (22 mg/dL), creatinine 100 μmol/L (1.1 mg/dL) and raised glucose at 56 mmol/L (1016 mg/dL). Her arterial blood gases showed a low pH of 7.05, low P_{CO_2} of 2.3 kPa (17.3 mmHg) and normal P_{O_2} of 13.0 kPa (97.7 mmHg).

• What is the cause of the volume depletion?

• What type of acid–base disturbance does she have?

• What is the underlying diagnosis and how should it be treated?

Case 10: A buried soldier with acute renal problems

A 24-year-old soldier from a bomb disposal unit was buried under rubble when a terrorist bomb exploded in a building that he was investigating. He was excavated from the rubble 18 h later by rescue workers and helicoptered to hospital. On arrival in hospital, he complained of pain in his left leg. On examination, he had multiple obvious minor injuries, but none to account for this pain. However, the muscles of his left leg and buttock were tender to palpation. He had passed only a small volume (20 mL) of dark-red urine since excavation.

His blood results were sodium 140 mmol/L, potassium 7.1 mmol/L, urea (BUN) 27 mmol/L (75.6 mg/dL), creatinine 580 μmol/L (6.6 mg/dL), creatine kinase 12 000 units/mL. His arterial pH was normal.

A cardiac monitor showed a sine wave pattern. Shortly after this was noted, he had a cardiac arrest. He was resuscitated and transferred to the intensive care unit.

• What is the cause of his renal failure?

• What was the cause of his cardiac arrest?

• What urgent treatment does he need to prevent a further cardiac arrest?

Case 11: Weakness and hypotension in a young man

A 24-year-old man presented with dizziness and weakness. He had a previous history of tuberculosis. On examination he was dehydrated and had a low blood pressure of 70/40. His blood results showed a plasma sodium of 125 mmol/L, potassium 6.0 mmol/L, creatinine 110 μmol/L (1.2 mg/dL), and glucose 3.0 mmol/L (54 mg/dL).

• What is the main circulating hormone controlling renal sodium excretion and how does it act?

• Can deficiency of this hormone account for the raised potassium level?

• What is the most likely diagnosis?

Case 12: A rash and renal problems

A 36-year-old woman presented with a cough productive of green sputum. She was treated with a course of ampicillin (a penicillin derivative). She re-presented 4 days later with a widespread rash over her arms and trunk. This was red, raised, and itchy. Her cough had improved and examination of her chest was normal.

On microscopy, her urine contained some eosinophils. Her full blood count showed a raised eosinophil level (20%) with a white cell count of 10×10^9 cells/L (10×10^3 cells/μL). Her plasma creatinine was 323 μmol/L (3.65 mg/dL)

• What is the likely cause of her raised plasma creatinine?

• What treatment might be helpful?

• What steps should be taken to prevent a similar problem in the future?

Case 1: A 10-year-old with generalized swelling

• This boy has nephrotic syndrome with heavy proteinuria (>3.5 g/24 h), hypoalbuminemia, and peripheral edema causing the swelling.

• In children, the most common cause of the nephrotic syndrome is minimal change nephropathy. This typically follows an upper respiratory infection and is more common in children with atopy (allergic eczema, asthma, and hay fever).

• Minimal change nephropathy responds well to steroids. Proteinuria usually resolves completely and does not leave permanent renal damage. If the disease does relapse, cyclosporin is sometimes used to prevent further relapse. See Chapters 30 and 33.

Case 2: A family history of hypertension and renal impairment

• The likely diagnosis is the autosomally dominant, inherited disorder of adult polycystic kidney disease. The features of this disease are hypertension, renal impairment, large kidneys, and often a family history of renal failure.

• Renal ultrasonography can easily confirm the diagnosis by demonstrating multiple cysts. Computed tomography or magnetic resonance imaging will also demonstrate the cysts.

• The prognosis is not good and progressive renal deterioration is likely. If his family members have developed end-stage renal disease, it is likely that he will as well. See Chapter 38.

Case 3: Colicky loin pain

• This pain is typical of renal colic caused by obstruction of the right ureter by a stone. If the stone is small, it should pass spontaneously. If it is large, intervention may be necessary.

• The presence of a stone can usually be confirmed by ultrasonography and, if the stone is radio-opaque, it may be seen on plain radiographs. Occasionally, it is necessary to inject radiocontrast dye into the collecting system to identify the site of the obstruction. This can be done through percutaneous puncture of the renal pelvis or by retrograde cannulation of the ureter through the urethra.

• The patient has a raised plasma calcium concentration and this can lead to hypercalciuria, which predisposes to calcium stone formation. There are many causes of hypercalcemia but, in an otherwise well patient, primary hyperparathyroidism is a possibility. This should be excluded by measurement of the plasma PTH level. See Chapters 24 and 47.

Case 4: An older man with nocturia and poor urinary flow

• The patient has clear symptoms of prostatic obstruction—poor flow, nocturia, hesitancy at the beginning, and dribbling at the end of micturition. He also has a palpable bladder after micturition, suggesting that he is not emptying his bladder properly during micturition. A rectal examination is essential to determine the size of the prostate and whether it feels hard and irregular, which would suggest prostate cancer.

• The urea and creatinine are raised because glomerular filtration is reduced. The cause of this is partial obstruction of the kidney due to reduced bladder outflow which is increasing the pressure in the urinary tract. This raised pressure is transmitted via the tubules to the glomerulus where it inhibits glomerular filtration.

• Measurement of the prostate-specific antigen (PSA) is helpful because, if it is raised significantly, this strongly suggests prostate cancer. See Chapters 40 and 48.

Case 5: Postoperative confusion in a young woman

• This patient has significant hyponatremia which is causing the confusion and lethargy.

• The hyponatremia is probably caused by intravenous administration of excess water in the form of 5% dextrose (glucose) solution. The dextrose is rapidly metabolized leaving only the water. Postoperatively, there is often excess antidiuretic hormone (ADH or vasopressin) secretion which promotes water retention. Hyponatremia in this setting can be symptomatic and serious in a young woman.

• The treatment is fluid restriction. If no further water is administered, the kidney will gradually excrete the excess. The condition is less common if the intravenous fluid used is predominantly isotonic 0.9% sodium chloride, rather than dextrose solution. See Chapters 18 and 19.

Case 6: Renal problems after vascular surgery

• The patient has acute renal failure with a rapid rise in plasma creatinine and a sudden fall in urine output. Several factors may contribute to postoperative renal failure. Hypotension during surgery can lead to renal ischemia and acute tubular necrosis. Renal ischemia can also arise from bleeding, inadequate volume replacement, or the undesirable hemodynamic effects of systemic infection. Postanaesthetic chest infections or lung collapse can cause hypoxia, which further contributes to renal ischemia. Nephrotoxic effects of drugs, particularly aminoglycosides such as gentamicin or non-steroidal anti-inflammatory drugs can cause renal impairment. In abdominal aortic aneurysm repair, a specific complication is damage to the renal arteries during the vascular surgery. In any abdominal surgery, damage to the ureters, although uncommon, can occur. They may be either ligated or transected.

• Renal angiography should demonstrate whether the renal arteries are intact and supplying the kidneys. Renal ultrasonography should reveal any obvious ligation or obstruction to the ureters. If these results are normal, the presumed diagnosis is acute tubular necrosis caused by the multiple factors mentioned above.

• Renal replacement is indicated if there is life-threatening hyperkalemia, metabolic acidosis, pulmonary edema, or severe uremic complications such as uremic pericarditis. See Chapter 40.

Case 7: Hypertension and renal impairment

• The patient is a smoker who has had a stroke. The bruits provide conclusive evidence that he has vascular disease. The abdominal bruits are consistent with renal artery stenosis, which could cause both the hypertension and the renal impairment.

• Renal angiography is currently the best investigation for making a clear-cut diagnosis of renal artery stenosis.

• Angiotensin II levels are high in renal artery stenosis. Angiotensin-converting enzyme inhibitors can cause a rapid deterioration in glomerular filtration rate in renal artery stenosis by blocking efferent arteriole vasoconstriction caused by angiotensin II. See Chapters 34 and 37.

Case 8: General malaise and itch with a pericardial rub

• The patient has presented with untreated chronic renal failure with symptoms and signs of the uremic syndrome, including malaise, itch, drowsiness, and evidence of pericarditis. The investigations show that both kidneys are small, consistent with chronic damage. In addition, she has anemia consistent with chronic erythropoietin deficiency. A low calcium can occur in acute or chronic renal failure, but is more characteristic of chronic renal failure.

• Factors that contribute to the hypocalcemia are a raised phosphate level caused by inadequate renal phosphate excretion and inadequate vitamin D synthesis by the failing kidney.

• PTH levels will be high. The low plasma calcium level stimulates PTH secretion (secondary hyperparathyroidism). Over time, the high PTH mobilizes calcium from bone and the plasma calcium rises. However, parathyroid cells can become autonomous and, even when calcium levels rise above normal, the PTH level may stay high (tertiary hyperparathyroidism). See Chapters 12, 24, 41, and 42.

Case 9: A young girl with thirst and rapid breathing

• A high plasma glucose level acts as an osmotic diuretic. The glucose is filtered freely and saturates tubular glucose reabsorption. The high tubular glucose concentration has an osmotic effect, which opposes water reabsorption and causes a diuresis and volume depletion. Volume depletion is manifest as a high pulse rate and postural hypotension (blood pressure that falls substantially on standing up).

• Her pH is low so she is acidotic. The P_{CO_2} is also low, which in itself would cause an alkalosis. This means that the low P_{CO_2} represents an attempt by the body to provide some respiratory compensation for the acidosis, which is therefore a metabolic acidosis.

• The underlying diagnosis is insulin-dependent (type 1) diabetes mellitus and she has acute diabetic ketoacidosis. Insulin deficiency allows a high glucose level to develop which causes the osmotic diuresis. In addition, in the absence of insulin, acidic ketones accumulate and cause the metabolic acidosis. These ketones provide a source of anions other than bicarbonate and chloride, and so the acidosis is an increased anion gap acidosis. Treatment is volume replacement with isotonic 0.9% saline solution. Insulin is given to lower plasma glucose by promoting glucose transport into cells and subsequent metabolism. Insulin also promotes metabolism of the acidic ketones. Insulin causes an intracellular movement of potassium and it may be necessary to administer potassium to prevent hypokalemia. See Chapters 22 and 26.

Case 10: A buried soldier with acute renal problems

• This patient has acute renal failure caused by rhabdomyolysis. His muscles were crushed by the rubble, and the pain and tenderness in his left leg and buttock are consistent with muscle injury. Damaged muscle releases potassium, creatine kinase, and myoglobin. Myoglobin colors the urine red and is a tubular toxin causing acute renal failure.

• He had life-threatening severe acute hyperkalemia. Acute hyperkalemia causes dangerous cardiac dysrhythmias. The typical ECG appearance of severe hyperkalemia is a sine wave appearance. This is a medical emergency and requires urgent treatment to prevent a cardiac arrest.

• Unfortunately, he did have a cardiac arrest. He was resuscitated, but his potassium level remains high, and he remains at risk of further cardiac arrest. He urgently requires hemodialysis or hemofiltration to remove the accumulated potassium. In the meantime, intravenous calcium can help to stabilize cardiac cell membranes and administration of insulin can promote a temporary intracellular shift of potassium. Glucose is usually given in addition to insulin to prevent hypoglycemia. In a hyperkalemic arrest intravenous calcium should always be administered. See Chapters 22 and 40.

Case 11: Weakness and hypotension in a young man

• Aldosterone is the main circulating hormone controlling renal sodium excretion. Aldosterone promotes distal tubular sodium reabsorption so aldosterone deficiency therefore causes renal sodium loss.

• Yes, aldosterone deficiency could account for the raised potassium level. In the principal cells of the distal tubule, sodium channels (ENaC) are activated by aldosterone. Influx of sodium ions into the cells can be thought of as promoting the activity of the basolateral Na^+/K^+ ATPase, which pumps potassium into the tubular cell. This potassium is then secreted through apical potassium channels. Deficiency of aldosterone reduces this potassium secretion causing hyperkalemia.

• There is hyponatremia, hyperkalemia, hypoglycemia, and volume depletion. The probable diagnosis is Addison's disease with aldosterone deficiency causing a low plasma sodium and a high plasma potassium. Excess sodium excretion carries water with it, causing volume depletion. Damage to the adrenal cortex, which produces aldosterone, can also reduce the production of glucocorticoids. Glucocorticoids maintain blood glucose levels, so glucocorticoid deficiency can cause hypoglycemia. The adrenal cortex can be destroyed by tuberculosis infection of the adrenal glands or by autoimmune processes. Damage by recurrent tuberculosis is the most probable cause of this patient's condition.

See Chapters 17, 18, 19, 21, and 22.

Case 12: A rash and renal problems

• It is likely that this patient has an acute interstitial nephritis. She has clearly had an allergic response to the antibiotic that she was given because she has a rash and eosinophilia. The renal equivalent of this rash is an acute interstitial nephritis, which can reduce glomerular filtration causing an elevated plasma creatinine. The eosinophils in the urine are consistent with an interstitial nephritis.

• The drug thought to be the cause of the interstitial nephritis, in this case the antibiotic, must be stopped. In addition, steroid therapy, usually with oral prednisolone, is generally helpful. The prognosis is usually good and full renal recovery is usual.

• It is important that the patient knows that she has had an allergic response to a specific drug and that this is clearly recorded in her medical notes. In future, she should not be given this drug again because the allergic effects are likely to recur. This should be explained to the patient.

See Chapter 32.

For further self-assessment visit *www.learndoctor.com.*

Index